Clinical Pharmacology of Selective Serotonin Reuptake Inhibitors

First Edition
Second Printing

Sheldon H. Preskorn, MD

Professor and Vice-Chairman,
Department of Psychiatry
University of Kansas School of Medicine–Wichita;
President and Medical Director,
Psychiatric Research Institute,
St. Francis Regional Medical Center,
Wichita, Kansas

Professional Communications, Inc.
A Publishing Corporation

Copyright 1996
Sheldon H. Preskorn, MD

Published by:
Professional Communications, **Inc**.

For orders only, please call:
1-800-337-9838

ISBN: 1-884735-08-8

Library of Congress Card Number: 95-071257

Printed in the United States of America

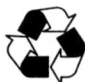

This text is printed on recycled paper.

ABOUT THE AUTHOR

Sheldon H. Preskorn, MD, is professor and vice-chairman, Department of Psychiatry, University of Kansas School of Medicine — Wichita. He is also the president and medical director of the Psychiatric Research Institute, Via Christi Health System in Wichita, Kansas.

An international lecturer and author of more than 200 scientific and professional articles, Dr Preskorn has received continuous grant funding since 1978 to allow him to conduct research primarily in the areas of psychopharmacology, affective and anxiety disorders, and neuroscience.

His basic pharmacological and neuroscience research has included studies in learning theory, neurochemistry, neurophysiology, histochemistry, electron microscopy, cerebral blood flow and metabolism, positron emission tomography, and radioligand binding. His clinical research has included pharmacokinetics and drug development through all clinical phases starting with "first-time-in-man" studies through registration proceedings.

Dr Preskorn has been a principal investigator during the clinical trial development programs of all eight antidepressants either marketed or recommended for approval in the US in the last 10 years. He has also been involved in the registration process of 7 out of these 8 drugs.

DEDICATION

To my wife, Belinda, and daughter, Erika, with love and gratitude for your understanding, patience and encouragement. To Wally and Marge. To all of my colleagues at the Psychiatric Research Institute and the University of Kansas School of Medicine, Department of Psychiatry — Wichita. To my patients. Thank you.

In memory of my parents, Harrison and Marie.

ACKNOWLEDGMENT

I gratefully acknowledge the patience, diligence and competence of my editor, Ms. Phyllis Jones Freeny. Without her, this book would not have become a reality. I also want to thank my secretary, Ms. Joyce Bishop, for her helpfulness and organizational skills.

Any miscues in this book are mine alone, but the people who contributed to and made possible the knowledge and insights contained in this book are legion. I want to, therefore, acknowledge and thank my mentors, colleagues, residents, medical students and patients, who have provided insights and intellectual stimulation throughout the years, with special thanks to: Annie Harvey, PhD; Dale Horst, PhD; David Greenblatt, MD; Elliott Richelson, MD; Richard Shader, MD; and, Lars Gram, MD.

TABBED TABLE OF CONTENTS

TABLES

viii

FIGURES

1 Introduction

Why have a book on selective serotonin reuptake inhibitors (SSRIs)? The rationale is simple: This class of antidepressants has become, for many physicians, the treatment of first choice for patients suffering from major depressive illness. The number of prescriptions for SSRIs in the United States equals that of the tricyclic antidepressants (TCAs), which were the gold standard antidepressants for almost 30 years. The widespread acceptance of SSRIs in the United States has occurred in a little over 7 years since the introduction of the SSRI, fluoxetine (Prozac). The introduction of this class has resulted in more than a four-fold increase in the antidepressant market in the United States because physicians are more willing to prescribe these medications to patients due to their greater safety and tolerability coupled with proven efficacy.

This handbook will provide a summary of the clinically relevant pharmacology of SSRIs in a manner that is "user friendly" for the practicing physician. The important similarities and differences will be presented, making liberal use of tables and figures to enhance the book's usefulness as a quick reference for the busy practitioner. The goal is to facilitate the optimum use of this important class of antidepressants.

Specific questions that this book will address include:

- How was this class of antidepressant drugs developed?
- What is the presumed mechanism of action (MOA) mediating their antidepressant efficacy?
- What accounts for their improved safety and tolerability relative to the old "gold standard" TCAs?

- What are the clinically meaningful differences among members of the SSRI class?
- What are the factors that the physician should consider when choosing a specific SSRI for a specific patient?

This book will provide a broad overview of the clinical pharmacology of SSRIs in terms of the similarities and differences between SSRIs and TCAs and between different members of the SSRI class. It will focus on studies that permit meaningful comparisons. It is not intended to focus only on the efficacy studies with these drugs, but rather to broadly examine their clinically relevant pharmacology. Since efficacy has been the focus of many other reviews of SSRIs, the data on this topic will be presented in a relatively brief summary form. This book will review how these drugs were developed, providing the foundation for understanding:

- Class differences between SSRIs and TCAs
- Class similarities between the SSRIs
- Pharmacokinetics of the SSRIs
- Effects of SSRIs on oxidative drug metabolism which are important to physicians since antidepressants are frequently used in combination with other medications by both psychiatric and nonpsychiatric physicians

Whenever possible, data on all five SSRIs marketed worldwide will be presented. However, comparable data does not exist for all the SSRIs on every issue addressed in this book. For example, fixed-dose studies have been published for fluoxetine, paroxetine and sertraline, but not for citalopram and fluvoxamine. In such instances, the data will be provided for the drugs that have published data. The omission and the reason for the omission of the other SSRIs will be noted at each appropriate place in the book.

2

Rational Drug Discovery and SSRIs

Over the past decade, tremendous strides have been made in the treatment of major depression due to the ability to rationally develop psychiatric medications.[215] In the last 10 years, 6 new medications have been marketed as antidepressants in the U.S. (Table 2.1):

- Bupropion
- Fluoxetine
- Sertraline
- Paroxetine
- Venlafaxine
- Nefazodone

Three of these drugs (fluoxetine, paroxetine and sertraline), together with two other drugs (citalopram and fluvoxamine) marketed as antidepressants elsewhere in the world, form the class known as selective serotonin reuptake inhibitors (SSRIs) (Figure 2.1). For many physicians, this class has supplanted tricyclic antidepressants (TCAs) as the antidepressant of first choice due to their greater safety and tolerabilty, coupled with comparable efficacy.

The rapid expansion in the number of antidepressants and the change in what is considered first-line therapy has been accompanied by a substantial amount of commercial claims and counterclaims. This situation can be confusing, even for physicians who specialize in clinical psychopharmacology, and even more so for the general physician who must also contend with developments in other therapeutic areas. Therefore, this book will explain the differences between

TABLE 2.1 — MAJOR CLASSES OF ANTIDEPRESSANTS DEFINED BY PRINCIPAL MECHANISMS OF ACTION

- Combined NE and 5-HT uptake inhibition, plus effects on multiple other neuroreceptors and fast sodium channels
  - Tertiary amine tricyclic antidepressants (TCAs)
- 5-HT uptake inhibition
  - Serotonin selective reuptake inhibitors (SSRIs)
- NE uptake inhibition
  - Secondary amine TCAs
- Combined NE and 5-HT uptake inhibition
  - Venlafaxine
- 5-HT2 receptor blockers and 5-HT uptake inhibition
  - Nefazodone (phenylpiperazine)
- DA and NE uptake inhibitors
  - Bupropion (aminoketones)
- Monoamine oxidase inhibitors (MAOIs)
  - Nonselective and irreversible
  - Selective and/or reversible (RIMAs)

the SSRIs and the TCAs, which were the mainstay of pharmacotherapy for major depression for many years, and discuss the clinically important similarities and differences between members of the SSRI class.

The development of SSRIs occurred over a relatively short interval of time. The first SSRI marketed was zimelidine by Astra. Unfortunately, several cases of Guillain-Barre syndrome were associated with the use of this drug and led to its withdrawal from the market. Nonetheless, five SSRIs were eventually launched successfully in multiple countries around the world. Each was developed by a different company:

- Citalopram by Lundbeck
- Fluvoxamine by Solvay
- Fluoxetine by Lilly
- Paroxetine by SmithKline-Beecham
- Sertraline by Pfizer

FIGURE 2.1— STRUCTURAL FORMULAS OF SEVERAL SSRIS

Citalopram

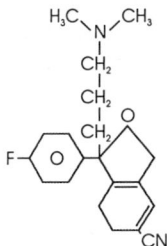

Fluoxetine

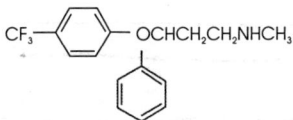

Fluvoxamine

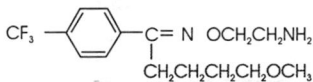

Paroxetine

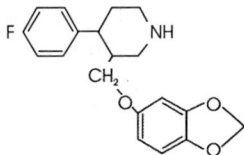

Sertraline

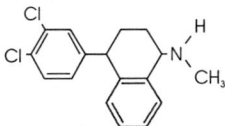

Parenthetically, while fluvoxamine is marketed as an antidepressant in many parts of the world, it is marketed only for obsessive-compulsive disorder in the U.S. Citalopram, while marketed in several countries in the world as an antidepressant, is not yet available in the U.S. Fluoxetine was the first SSRI marketed in the United States in 1988. Table 10.2 (in the Appendix) lists the SSRIs that are available in various countries.

The fact that the five SSRIs were produced by five different companies is a testimony to the shift from a discovery process dependent on chance observation to a process of rational drug development. Understanding rational drug development is pivotal to understanding the clinical pharmacology of SSRIs.

How the SSRIs were developed is a scientific success story. The SSRIs are the first rationally designed class of psychotropic medications and, hence, have launched a new era in psychotropic drug development. The strategy behind rational drug development is to design a new drug that is capable of affecting a specific neural site of action (SOA) (eg, uptake pumps, receptors) while avoiding effects on other SOAs. The goal in such development is to produce agents that are more efficacious, safer and better tolerated than older medications (Table 2.2).[215] This enhanced safety profile includes a reduced likelihood of pharmaco-dynamically mediated adverse drug-drug interactions by avoiding affects on SOAs that are not essential to the intended outcome (eg, antidepressant efficacy).

A few general comments about what a drug must do to produce a specific clinical effect may be helpful to put this book in perspective. A drug must act on an SOA that is physiologically relevant to the effect (Figure 2.2). That SOA may be, by way of example but not limited to, an uptake pump, an enzyme, or a receptor. The drug "recognizes" and binds to that SOA. The activation or inhibition of a specific site is termed

18

TABLE 2.2 — CRITERIA FOR NEW DRUG DEVELOPMENT

- *Inclusion criteria*: have the desired MOA
- *Exclusion criteria*: avoid effects of other MOAs

Goals of Such Development

- Maintain or enhance efficacy
- Increase therapeutic index
- Improve tolerability profile
- Reduce likelihood of pharmacodynamic drug-drug interactions

Reference: 217

FIGURE 2.2— SCHEMATIC ILLUSTRATION OF RELATIONSHIP BETWEEN DRUG SITE OF ACTION AND EFFECT

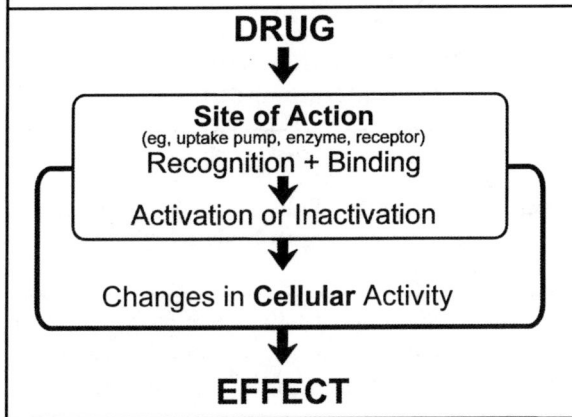

DRUG

↓

Site of Action
(eg, uptake pump, enzyme, receptor)
Recognition + Binding

↓

Activation or Inactivation

↓

Changes in **Cellular** Activity

↓

EFFECT

the drug's mechanism of action (MOA). For example, a drug may be an agonist or antagonist at a specific serotonin receptor.

A given drug may affect one or more SOAs over its clinically relevant dosing range and, therefore, may produce multiple and different clinical effects, some desired and some not. Drugs that affect multiple SOAs are more characteristic of drugs developed based on chance discovery, whereas the goal of rational drug development is to produce drugs with a more limited range of effects (Table 2.2).

Prior to the SSRIs, all psychotropic medications were the result of chance observation (Table 2.3). Lithium came from studies looking for putative endogenous psychomimetic substances excreted in the urine of psychotic patients.[51] The phenothiazines came from a search for better preanesthetic agents.[154] The TCAs were the result of an unsuccessful attempt to improve on the antipsychotic effectiveness of phenothiazines.[148] The monoamine oxidase inhibitors (MAOIs) came from a failed attempt to develop effective antitubercular medications.[63] The first studies of benzodiazepines were unsuccessful attempts to treat patients with schizophrenia.

TABLE 2.3 — THE EVOLUTION OF PSYCHOPHARMACOLOGY

- First generation discovered by chance (eg, tricyclic antidepressants)
- Advanced generations discovered by design based on molecular targeting (eg, serotonin selective reuptake inhibitors)

Despite these initial failed attempts to use these various drugs therapeutically, astute clinical investigators recognized their therapeutic value in other conditions: lithium for manic-depression, phenothiazines for psychotic disorders, TCAs and MAOIs for major depression, and benzodiazepines for anxiety disorders.

This chance discovery process is not unique to psychiatry, but instead has been the universal first step in any therapeutic area.[210] Prior to such first steps, too little knowledge of the biology underlying illnesses existed to permit a more rational approach to drug development. However, these first drugs played an important role in providing the first insights into the pathophysiology underlying the illness or, at least, underlying drug responsiveness.

Molecular targeting is the essence of rational drug development.[211] In this approach, the specific target(s) of interest is a fundamental brain mechanism believed to be important in the pathophysiology underlying a specific psychopathologic condition or psychiatric syndrome (eg, major depression). This SOA may be the neuronal uptake pump for a neurotransmitter, a specific neurotransmitter receptor subtype, or a subunit of an ion channel (Figure 2.2).

As was the case with each of the SSRIs, the new molecular entity is developed to stereospecifically interact with the target of interest. At the same time, the molecule is structurally modified so that it does not interact with other targets that mediate unwanted effects (eg, peripheral anticholinergic effects). Through this systematic approach, a new candidate drug is selected for clinical testing to support registration for marketing. This type of rational drug development is now possible in psychiatry because of the improved understanding of central and peripheral mechanisms of action (MOAs) relevant to both desired and undesired central and peripheral effects.

Antidepressant pharmacotherapy is the first area in psychopharmacology to have benefitted significantly from such targeted development.[215] Figure 2.3 illustrates the evolution of antidepressants over the past three decades. TCAs and MAOIs were the first successful antidepressants, but their antidepressant properties were discovered by chance, as discussed above. Nonetheless, this chance discovery was important. First, these drugs provided the first scientifically proven treatments for major depression and demonstrated that major depression was amenable to medi-

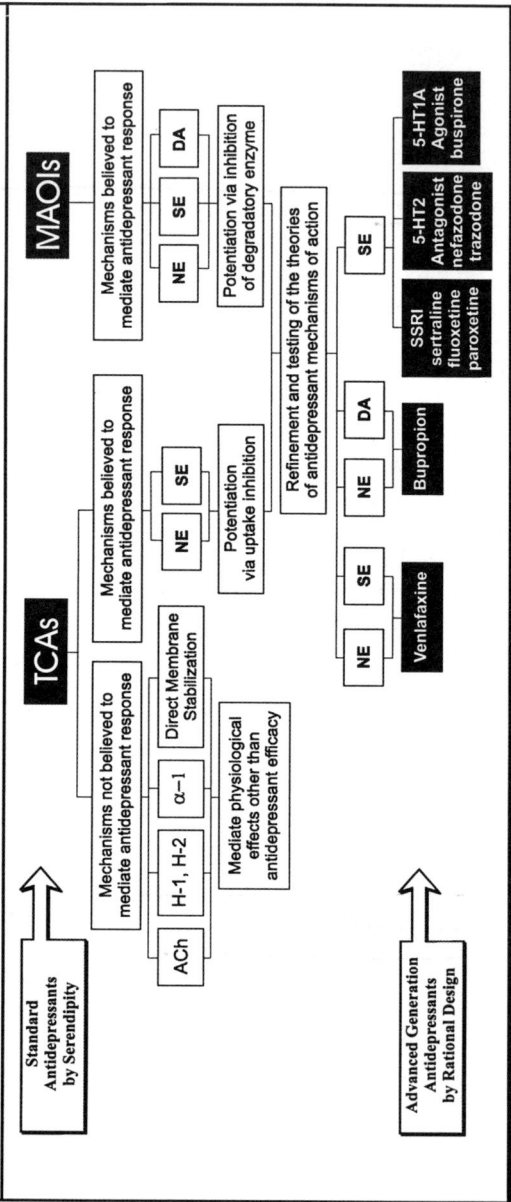

FIGURE 2.3 — STANDARD AND NEW GENERATION ANTIDEPRESSANTS MECHANISMS OF ACTION

cal intervention just as other medical conditions, such as hypertension and diabetes. Second, they served as roadmaps to improve our understanding of the MOAs, mediating both their desired antidepressant effects and undesired effects. This information was critical to the rational drug development efforts that followed and led to the SSRIs and other new antidepressants.

2

In the case of major depression, TCAs and MAOIs implicated the potentiation of neurotransmission in one or more than one central biogenic amine neural system as potential MOAs responsible for their antidepressant efficacy. That finding, coupled with improved means of isolating and studying the effects of drugs on specific neural mechanisms, led to the development of the SSRIs.

The nature of older chance-discovery drugs is that they have many clinical effects either because they affect an SOA with broad implications for organ function (eg, MAOIs that affect an enzyme responsible for the degradation of four major neurotransmitters) or because they affect multiple SOAs (eg, TCAs). Such drugs typically have:

- Narrow therapeutic indices
- Poor tolerability profiles
- Potential for causing multiple types of pharmacodynamic interactions with a wide variety of concomitantly prescribed medications

The SSRIs were developed based on the knowledge gained from studying the effects of the TCAs and the techniques developed in basic neuroscience research to isolate and study the effects of drugs on specific neural SOAs (eg, uptake pumps, receptors). In the case of the SSRIs, each was the product of a similar development strategy in which the goal was to produce a drug capable of inhibiting the neuronal uptake pump for serotonin, a property shared with the TCAs, but without affecting the various other neuroreceptors (ie, histamine, acetylcholine, and α-adrenergic receptors) or fast sodium channels, affected by the TCAs. Actions on these latter sites are responsible for many of the safety and tolerability problems of the TCAs.[220,221] The fact that SSRIs were designed to avoid affecting these other SOAs explains many of the pharmacological differences between the SSRIs and the TCAs (see Section 4) and explains the similarities among the SSRIs (see Section 5). In many ways, the SSRIs are to psychiatry as β-blockers are to internal medicine.

In contrast to rational development, chance discovery is usually dependent on the drug's having a large signal-to-noise ratio (ie, a big clinical effect or multiple clinical effects). Unfortunately, this fact means that chance-discovery drugs typically will produce a number of undesired, as well as desired, effects and will have a narrower therapeutic index in comparison with a drug that was rationally developed to affect only the SOA(s) necessary to produce the desired response.

This issue can be readily understood by examining the pharmacology of TCAs that has served as the cornerstone of antidepressant pharmacotherapy for almost 30 years. TCAs affect multiple SOAs over a relatively narrow concentration range so that patients are likely to experience multiple effects while taking these medications.[34,66,221,225] Some MOAs of TCAs (ie, the inhibition of the fast sodium channels) can cause potentially serious effects on cardiac conduction and occur at concentrations only an order of magnitude higher than the concentration needed to inhibit the neuronal uptake pumps for norepinephrine and serotonin, the putative MOAs mediating the antidepressant effects of TCAs. This fact explains why an overdose of TCAs of only 5 to 10 times their therapeutic dose can cause serious toxicity and why patients who have a slow clearance rate for these drugs can develop serious ad-

24

verse effects on routine doses due to the accumulation of toxic concentrations.[228]

To put this issue with TCAs in perspective, Table 2.4 illustrates the cocktail of drugs, each having only one predominant MOA, that would have to be given to a patient to reproduce the effects that occur in a patient receiving a tertiary amine TCA, such as amitriptyline. Obviously, the problem with amitriptyline is that the patient has to experience a large number of effects to receive the benefit of the mechanism that mediates antidepressant response.

The issue of multiple MOAs over a narrow concentration range is further complicated by the fact that there is a large interindividual variability in the clearance rates of TCAs, even in physically healthy individuals.[213] The variability is even larger when dealing with the elderly, the medically ill, and patients on con-

TABLE 2.4 — TCA (AMITRIPTYLINE) POLYPHARMACY IN A SINGLE PILL

Drug	Action
Chlorpheniramine	Histamine-1 receptor blockade
Cimetidine	Histamine-2 receptor blockade
Benztropine	Acetylcholine receptor blockade
Desipramine	Norepinephrine uptake inhibition
Sertraline	Serotonin uptake inhibition
Nefazodone	5-HT2 receptor blockade
Prazosin	NE-α_1 receptor blockade
Yohimbine	NE-α_2 receptor blockade
Quinidine	Direct membrane stabilization

The multiple actions of amitriptyline are listed in descending order of potency (ie, histamine-1 receptor blockade is the most potent, whereas direct membrane stabilization is the least.)

comitant medications that can either induce or inhibit the clearance of these drugs. With TCAs, patients can have numerous types of adverse effects ranging from nuisance problems (eg, dry mouth) to serious toxicity (eg, seizures, cardiac arrhythmias). Patients who clear the drugs slowly may experience the latter due to the accumulation of excessive concentrations despite being on conventional doses.

This situation is made even more complicated because the early signs of TCA-induced toxicity can mimic worsening of major depression so that the physician may unfortunately respond by increasing rather than reducing the dose.[227] These facts considered together have made therapeutic drug monitoring (TDM), at least once during early treatment (at the end of the first week of treatment with a stable dose), a standard aspect when prescribing TCAs.[221,228] Using the TDM results, rational dose adjustment can then be made to compensate for the intraindividual differences in clearance rate, and thus ensure that the patient will be treated with a dose that will achieve a concentration that is optimal for most patients with regard to efficacy, safety and cost effectiveness.

Unfortunately, TDM-driven dose adjustment does not substantially improve the tolerability of TCAs because MOAs for producing adverse effects (eg, those mediated by histamine or muscarinic receptor blockade) are more potent and hence occur at lower concentrations than their presumed MOAs underlying their antidepressant efficacy (ie, inhibiting the neuronal uptake for norepinephrine and serotonin) (Figure 2.4). Hence, patients who are sensitive to a given MOA may experience discomforting adverse effects even at concentrations that are subtherapeutic for treating major depression. That problem has been addressed by rational drug development of new drugs (eg, SSRIs) with a much wider gap between their potency for an effect on the desired versus undesired targets. As a result,

26

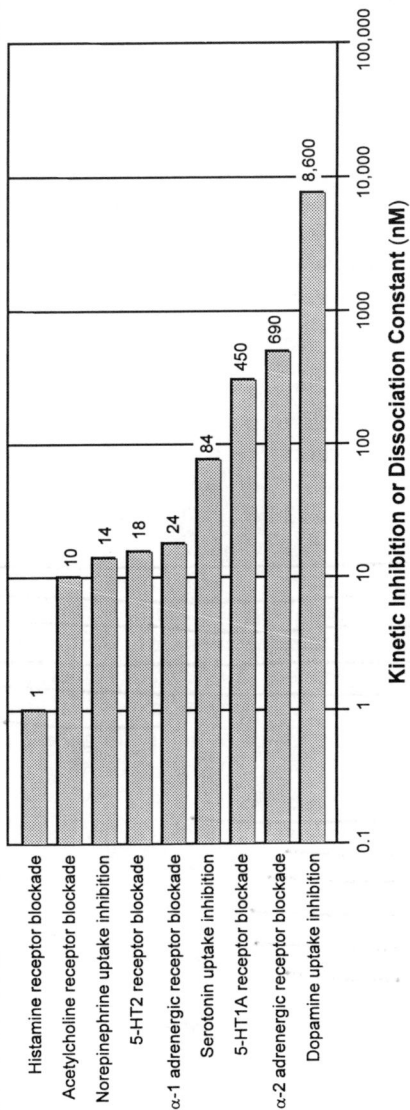

FIGURE 2.4 — *IN VITRO* POTENCY OF AMITRIPTYLINE AS A REPRESENTATIVE TRICYCLIC ANTIDEPRESSANT FOR DIFFERENT SITES OF ACTION AND RELATED MECHANISMS OF ACTION

Site of action	Kinetic Inhibition or Dissociation Constant (nM)
Histamine receptor blockade	1
Acetylcholine receptor blockade	10
Norepinephrine uptake inhibition	14
5-HT2 receptor blockade	18
α-1 adrenergic receptor blockade	24
Serotonin uptake inhibition	84
5-HT1A receptor blockade	450
α-2 adrenergic receptor blockade	690
Dopamine uptake inhibition	8,600

Adapted from references: 34, 66

we now have seven major classes of antidepressants based on putative MOAs mediating antidepressant response (Table 2.1).

The SSRIs were all developed to have a similar MOA: the potentiation of serotonin (5-HT) by the inhibition of its neuronal uptake pump. As such, all SSRIs have common 5-HT agonistic effects that appear to mediate both their desired (eg, antidepressant efficacy) and undesired (eg, sexual dysfunction) reactions. As a class, SSRIs are considerably more selective in comparison to TCAs in terms of their central nervous system MOAs, but differ in other clinically important ways, as will be discussed in detail in this book (see Sections 6 through 8).

The reason to choose serotonin uptake inhibition as the desired MOA is based on the emerging understanding of the role of serotonin in the brain as well as on the pharmacology of TCAs and MAOIs. From a phylogenetic standpoint, serotonin is one of the oldest neurotransmitters.[255] It is found in such relatively simple organisms as jellyfish. In the human brain, serotonin-containing neurons are highly localized in specific clusters in the brainstem and spinal cord.[271] From these sites, the cells send out axons that end in serotonin-containing terminals innervating the diverse areas throughout the brain. These regions include:

- Spinothalamic pain fibers
- Brainstem
- Cerebellum
- Hypothalamus
- Basal ganglia
- Neocortex

This anatomy explains why serotonin is implicated in so many brain functions including:

- Pain perception
- Sleep
- Thermal regulation

28

- Appetite
- Gut regulation
- Balance
- Reproductive function
- Motor function
- Higher cognitive function
- Sensory interpretation

Given these diverse responsibilities, dysfunction of serotonin neurons have been implicated in a wide variety of diseases, including major depression. For the same reason, serotonin-active drugs can have many different clinical effects by virtue of their physiological effects on diverse brain regions. This anatomy explains why even "selective" drugs such as SSRIs can produce so many diverse clinical effects (eg, nausea, a feeling of incoordination, suppression of REM sleep, decreased libido, akathisia) as well as being useful in such apparently disparate disorders as major depression, anxiety disorders, pain disorders, and premature ejaculation. While SSRIs are "selective" in terms of affecting the neuronal uptake pump for serotonin, this action affects a multitude of specific postsynaptic serotonin receptors (eg, 5-HT1A, 5-HT1D, 5-HT2A, 5-HT2C, and 5-HT3) which, in turn, affects a multitude of neural systems.[128]

Chirality

Although all SSRIs are products of rational drug development, one of the major goals of such a development was not realized with two of the SSRIs due to the phenomenon of chirality: that goal was to produce a drug that is a single molecule with a precise, limited (or focused) range of pharmacological actions. If the molecule has an asymmetrical carbon, then it exists in enantiomeric forms (ie, chirality). As can be seen in Figure 2.1, all of the SSRIs except fluvoxamine have an asymmetrical carbon. However, only one enantiomer of paroxetine and sertraline, respectively, is contained in the marketed formulation of these two drugs. In contrast, citalopram and fluoxetine are marketed as the racemates of their two enantiomers. Hence, patients on these two SSRIs achieve plasma and tissue levels of each enantiomer and their respective metabolites, which are also enantiomers.

This fact raises the question of whether there are substantial differences in the pharmacodynamics and pharmacokinetics of these enantiomers and whether such differences contribute in a meaningful way to the variance in drug response among different patients.[12] If the different enantiomers have meaningful differences in their therapeutic ratios, one enantiomer can contribute disproportionately to adverse consequences relative to therapeutic benefit. The presence of enantiomers complicates the use of TDM in both research and clinical practice since many assays will not distinguish between the two enantiomeric forms of a drug. If there are meaningful differences in their pharmacodynamics and pharmacokinetics, that fact can add substantial "noise" to such results and thus confound their interpretation.

As is the case with the enantiomers of citalopram and fluoxetine, there is often limited data on their relative pharmacodynamics and pharmacokinetics to answer these questions. A summary of that data for these two SSRIs follows.

The racemic mixture of citalopram produces racemic desmethylcitalopram and didesmethylcitalopram. The S-enantiomers are potent and selective inhibitors of serotonin uptake in contrast to the relatively inactive corresponding R-enantiomers.[130] The active S-enantiomer of citalopram is generally only one-third of the total citalopram plasma level under steady-state conditions.[242] However, there is variability in this ratio among different patients that may be characteristic of patients genetically deficient in cytochrome P450 (CYP) 2C19.[242] CYP 2C19 enzyme is the principal enzyme responsible for the metabolism of citalopram.[254]

This variability in the ratio of the active to the relatively inactive enantiomer can contribute to variability in response to the drug among different patients. Given the relative levels and activity of the enantiomers of citalopram and its metabolites, studies attempting to correlate plasma levels of citalopram with serotonin mediated effects should report on the levels of each enantiomer or should focus on the levels of S-citalopram.

Racemic fluoxetine produces racemic norfluoxetine. While S-fluoxetine, R-fluoxetine, and S-norfluoxetine are potent and selective inhibitors of serotonin uptake *in vitro* and *in vivo*, that is not true for R-norfluoxetine.[98,290,291] Under steady-state conditions, the plasma levels of racemic fluoxetine and norfluoxetine are comparable.[189] Thus, studies attempting to correlate the plasma levels of fluoxetine and norfluoxetine should ideally take into account the relative inactivity of the R-norfluoxetine in terms of the inhibition of serotonin uptake.

The R-enantiomers of fluoxetine and norfluoxetine are also weaker inhibitors of CYP 2D6 than are the S-enantiomers.[267] Thus, failure to distinguish between these enantiomers in studies attempting to correlate plasma levels of fluoxetine and norfluoxetine with the inhibition of the metabolism of CYP 2D6-dependent substrates will hamper the ability to establish such a relationship.

Tables summarizing the above data are found in the sections dealing with the effects of the SSRIs on neural mechanisms (Section 3, Table 3.4) and on CYP enzymes (Section 8, Table 8.11), respectively. There may be other important differences in the pharmacodynamics and pharmacokinetics of the enantiomers of these two SSRIs which are not known at this time. There is little active research ongoing in this area; therefore, knowledge of these enantiomers may not expand appreciably in the near future. This discussion should be kept in mind as a caveat when reading the rest of this book. Unless specified otherwise, the data in this book on *in vitro* and *in vivo* studies with citalopram and fluoxetine were done with the racemic mixtures, and the plasma and tissue levels reported of the parent compound and the metabolites are the combined levels of their enantiomeric forms.

3 Basic Neuropharmacology of SSRIs

Potency and selectivity are fundamental pharmacological concepts essential to understanding the basic neuropharmacology and the clinical psychopharmacology of serotonin selective reuptake inhibitors (SSRIs) including:

- Why SSRIs differ so much from the tricyclic antidepressants (TCAs)
- Why SSRIs are so similar in terms of their psychiatric effects

In this section, we will:

- Review results from several studies that examine the *in vitro* binding affinities of SSRIs and their major metabolites for clinically important neural receptors and uptake pumps (ie, sites of action [SOAs])
- Contrast these binding affinities with those of clomipramine and its major metabolite, desmethylclomipramine, to illustrate the basic pharmacological differences between the TCAs and the SSRIs

How *In Vitro* Studies Are Done to Determine Potency

As discussed in Section 2, the goal in developing the SSRIs is to design drugs capable of inhibiting the neuronal uptake pump for serotonin as with the TCAs, but at the same time, avoiding actions on other neural mechanisms. The first step involves isolating these neural SOAs so that the effects of drugs on them can

33

be studied *in vitro*.[34,129] One approach is to isolate the neuronal uptake pump for serotonin by homogenizing brain regions rich in serotonin terminal fields. The homogenization process lysises the neuronal membranes in such a way that the membrane can close back on itself to form synaptosome preparations which retain the functional integrity of the serotonin uptake pump. The pumps allow the synaptosomes to concentrate serotonin by taking it up from the fluid in which the synaptosomes are suspended. By radioactively tagging the serotonin, the rate of uptake can measure by adding tagged serotonin to the suspension for a specified period of time, then centrifuging and counting radioactivity in the synaptosomal pellet and expressing the result as the amount of radioactivity per milligram of protein. The ability of different drugs to slow or inhibit the pump can then be studied by adding different concentrations of a specific drug to identical aliquots of the same synaptosomal preparation and studying ability of the synaptosomal preparation to take up radioactive serotonin as a function of the concentration of the inhibitor which has been added. All other variables, besides the amount of inhibitor added, are kept the same among the different aliquots.

The results from such a study are plotted in Figure 3.1 as a classic concentration-response curve in which the Y-axis is the response (ie, effect of the drug) and the X-axis is increasing concentration of the investigational drug (ie, the potential inhibitor). In the case of the serotonin uptake pump, the effect is the degree of slowing or inhibition of the uptake of the radioactive serotonin into the synaptosomes. This approach represents a biological assay of the effect of the drug on its SOA rather than simply the binding affinity of the drug for the SOA.

FIGURE 3.1 — GENERIC CURVE OF A DRUG'S CONCENTRATION-DEPENDENT EFFECT ON SPECIFIC SOA*

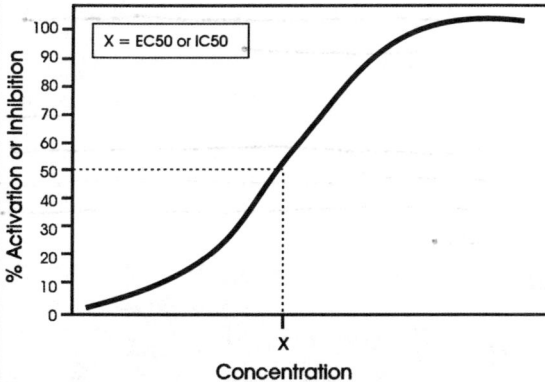

X = EC50 or IC50

% Activation or Inhibition

Concentration

* The effect (ie, activation or inhibition) of the drug on the site of action (SOA) is the drug's mechanism of action (MOA).

In another version of Figure 3.1, the Y-axis can be the binding affinity of the drug for a specific SOA (eg, the histamine$_1$ receptor) rather than its effect on the site.[66] In this case, the affinity of the drug for a receptor is measured by its ability to displace a radioactive tagged ligand. From a binding assay, one cannot tell whether the drug is an agonist or an antagonist at that specific SOA; instead, only the affinity of the drug for the receptor is determined.

In either approach, the inflection point is a reproducible measure of the drug's affinity for the site or its effect on the site and hence can be used for comparison purposes across different drugs (ie, relative *in vitro* potency for that SOA).

As discussed in Section 2, such studies have been done as part of the development process of all of the SSRIs to determine what chemical structure will:

- Convey high affinity for the serotonin uptake pump
- Slow or inhibit the pump when it bound to it
- Have low affinity for the multiple neuro-receptors known to be responsible for many of the adverse effects of the TCAs (eg, acetyl-choline, histamine, and adrenergic receptors)
- Not inhibit fast sodium channels which cause the cardiotoxicity problems associated with TCAs

Results of *In Vitro* Studies Done on the Effects of Different SSRIs on Different Biogenic Amine Uptake Pumps

Tables 3.1, 3.2 and 3.3 show the results from three different *in vitro* studies comparing the effects of four representative TCAs and all five SSRIs on the neuronal uptake pumps for serotonin, norepinephrine and dopamine. As can be seen, the SSRIs are all more potent inhibitors of serotonin uptake than are the TCAs, with the exception of clomipramine, which is less potent than paroxetine or sertraline, approximately equal to citalopram, and more potent than fluoxetine or fluvoxamine.

The results from the three studies also illustrate the variability that can be obtained in terms of rank order, particularly when the drugs are relatively close in potency. In Study 1, sertraline is approximately twice as potent as paroxetine, whereas in the other two studies, paroxetine is 2- to 5-times more potent than sertraline. Therefore, the rank order shown on the bottom half of the table can change somewhat from one study to the next.

TABLE 3.1 — EFFECT OF ANTIDEPRESSANTS ON SEROTONIN UPTAKE *IN VITRO**

Drug	Study 1[1]	Study 2[2]	Study 3[3]
Sertraline	0.19	0.85	3.40
Paroxetine	0.29	0.44	0.73
Clomipramine	1.50	2.25	—
Citalopram	1.80	2.71	—
Fluvoxamine	3.80	3.08	—
Fluoxetine	6.8	87.0	93.0
Imipramine	35.00	31.80	41.00
Amitriptyline	39.00	67.20	84.00
Desipramine	200.00	182.00	180.00
Relative Potency of Antidepressant on 5-HT Uptake *In Vitro*[†]			
Drug	Study 1[1]	Study 2[2]	Study 3[3]
Sertraline	1.0	2.0	4.7
Paroxetine	1.5	1.0	1.0
Clomipramine	8.0	5.0	—
Citalopram	10.0	6.0	—
Fluvoxamine	20.0	7.0	—
Fluoxetine	36.0	25.0	19.0
Imipramine	184.0	95.0	56.0
Amitriptyline	205.0	153.0	115.0
Desipramine	1,053.0	414.0	247.0

* IC50 values (nM); rat brain tissues for Studies 1 and 2 and kinetic inhibition constant (K_i) for Study 3.

† Determined by dividing the IC50 for each drug by the IC50 for the most potent drug in each study. The lower the number, the greater the potency.

References: [1]129, [2]250, [3]34

TABLE 3.2 — EFFECT OF ANTIDEPRESSANTS ON NOREPINEPHRINE UPTAKE *IN VITRO**

Drug	Study 1[1]	Study 2[2]	Study 3[3]
Sertraline	160.00	159.00	220.00
Paroxetine	81.00	22.20	33.00
Clomipramine	21.00	14.60	—
Citalopram	6,100.00	2,750.00	—
Fluvoxamine	620.00	299.00	—
Fluoxetine	370.00	85.30	143.00
Imipramine	14.00	12.00	14.00
Amitriptyline	24.00	14.20	13.90
Desipramine	0.83	0.65	0.61

Relative Potency of Antidepressant on Norepinephrine Uptake *In Vitro*[†]

Drug	Study 1[1]	Study 2[2]	Study 3[3]
Sertraline	193.0	245.0	360.0
Paroxetine	98.0	34.0	54.0
Clomipramine	25.0	22.0	—
Citalopram	7,349.0	4,231.0	—
Fluvoxamine	747.0	460.0	—
Fluoxetine	446.0	131.0	234.0
Imipramine	17.0	18.0	23.0
Amitriptyline	29.0	22.0	21.0
Desipramine	1.0	1.0	1.0

* IC50 values (nM); rat brain tissues for Studies 1 and 2 and kinetic inhibition constant (K_i) for Study 3.

† Determined by dividing the IC50 for each drug by the IC50 for the most potent drug in each study. The lower the number, the greater the potency.

References: [1]129, [2]250, [3]34

TABLE 3.3 — EFFECT OF ANTIDEPRESSANTS ON DOPAMINE UPTAKE *IN VITRO**

Drug	Study 1[1]	Study 2[2]	Study 3[3]
Sertraline	48	78	260
Paroxetine	5,100	540	1,700
Clomipramine	4,300	3,810	—
Citalopram	40,000	> 10,000	—
Fluvoxamine	42,000	10,000	—
Fluoxetine	5,000	3,160	3,050
Imipramine	17,000	10,000	11,000
Amitriptyline	5,300	> 10,000	8,600
Desipramine	9,100	6,530	11,000
Relative Potency of Antidepressant on Dopamine Uptake *In Vitro*†			
Drug	Study 1[1]	Study 2[2]	Study 3[3]
Sertraline	1	1	1
Paroxetine	106	7	7
Clomipramine	90	49	—
Citalopram	830	> 125	—
Fluvoxamine	875	> 125	—
Fluoxetine	104	41	12
Imipramine	350	> 125	141
Amitriptyline	110	> 125	110
Desipramine	190	84	141

* IC50 values (nM); rat brain tissues for Studies 1 and 2 and kinetic inhibition constant (K_i) for Study 3.
† Determined by dividing the IC50 for each drug by the IC50 for the most potent drug in each study. The lower the number, the greater the potency.

References: [1]129, [2]250, [3]34

Nonetheless, SSRIs are all substantially more potent in terms of their affinity for the serotonin pump compared with their affinity for or action on any other neurotransmitter pumps or neuroreceptors. When drugs are this selective, differences in potency after a point become clinically irrelevant since the concentration can be adjusted to achieve inhibition of the desired target without affecting any other target. This fact is the essence of the concept of pharmacological selectivity (Figure 3.2).

In Table 3.2, the results for the same drugs from the same studies are shown with regard to their inhibition of the norepinephrine reuptake pump. As can readily be seen, the TCAs are substantially more potent with regard to this action in comparison to all of the SSRIs. As shown on the bottom half, all the SSRIs are two to three orders of magnitude less potent than is the TCA, desipramine, in terms of the ability to inhibit the norepinephrine uptake pump.

In Table 3.3, results are shown for the inhibition of the dopamine uptake pump. None of the TCAs or the SSRIs have substantial action on this neurotransmitter pump. Although sertraline is consistently the most potent, it is still 100 times less potent in terms of inhibiting the dopamine versus the serotonin uptake pump. That means the physician would have to increase the dose (ie, the concentration) of sertraline 100 times higher than that needed to inhibit the serotonin uptake pump before a comparable effect would be achieved on the dopamine uptake pump. Thus, the ratios shown in the bottom of Table 3.3 can be misleading if not viewed within the context of the actual affinity of the drug for a secondary SOA relative to its affinity for its primary SOA and relative to the clinically relevant concentration needed to produce the desired clinical effect. Recall that citalopram and fluoxetine are marketed as racemates (see Section 2). The values shown in the above tables for uptake inhi-

40

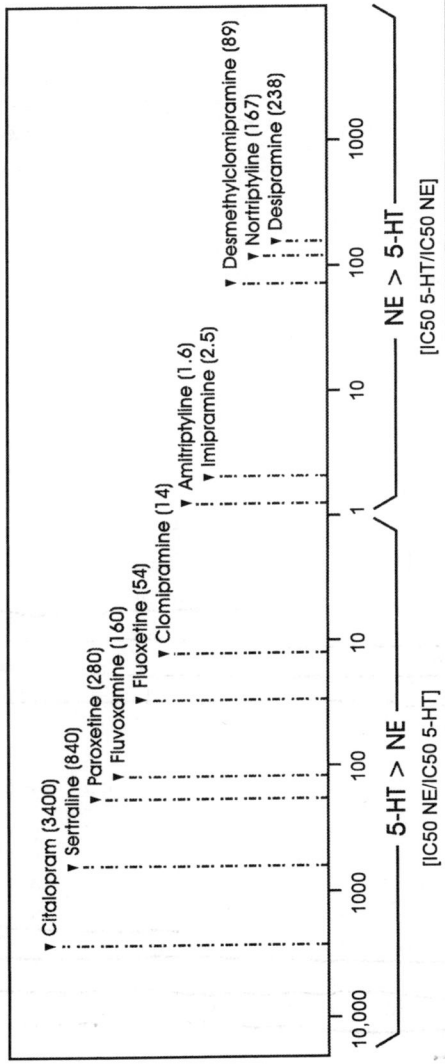

FIGURE 3.2 — SELECTIVITY RATIOS FOR A SERIES OF UPTAKE INHIBITORS MEASURED *IN VITRO*

Data from reference: 129

41

bition are for the racemates of these two SSRIs. Table 3.4 shows the value for the individual enantiomers of each of these SSRIs and their major metabolite.

The Concept of Selectivity as Related to Effects on Different Biogenic Amine Uptake Pumps

The concept of selectivity is further illustrated in Table 3.5. In this table, the affinity of a specific drug for the norepinephrine uptake pump is divided by its affinity for the serotonin uptake pump. As seen in Tables 3.1, 3.2 and 3.3, the more potent a drug, the smaller the concentration needed to affect or bind to an SOA. Thus, the less potent effect is a larger number (ie, more concentration is needed to produce the same degree of effect), and the more potent effect is the smaller number. In Table 3.5, the ratio is appreciably greater than "1" for all SSRIs, whereas the ratio for all TCAs, except clomipramine, is considerably smaller than "1." SSRIs are considerably more potent at inhibiting the serotonin uptake pump than the norepinephrine uptake pump, whereas the opposite is true for the TCAs, with the exception of clomipramine.

The more the ratio diverges from "1" in either direction, the more selective the drug is for one pump over the other. For example, all SSRIs, with the exception of fluoxetine, are more than 100 times more potent at inhibiting the serotonin versus the norepinephrine uptake pump, whereas the converse is true for the TCA, desipramine. A concentration of any SSRI that will produce substantial inhibition of the serotonin uptake pump will produce no physiologically meaningful inhibition of the norepinephrine uptake pump. The converse will be true for TCAs such as desipramine. Clinically, such selectivity ratios translate into being able to produce all the physiological effects mediated by inhibiting one pump without causing any effects that will be produced by inhibiting the other uptake pump.

Figure 3.2 graphically illustrates the same point. In this figure, a value of "1" means that the drug will inhibit both uptake pumps at the same concentration (ie, no selectivity with regard to effect on these two SOAs). For illustration purposes, the ratio of the right side of the figure is the potency for inhibiting the uptake of serotonin divided by the potency for inhibiting the uptake for norepinephrine, while the inverse is demonstrated on the left side of the figure. This approach is taken so that the ratios will become larger in either direction and hence may be intuitively simpler to understand. In this figure, desipramine is 238 times more potent at inhibiting the norepinephrine uptake pump versus the serotonin uptake pump, whereas all the SSRIs, with the exception of fluoxetine, are over 100 times more potent at inhibiting the serotonin versus the norepinephrine uptake pump.

Affecting any SOA can cause adverse as well as beneficial effects. The physiological responses mediated by activation or inhibition of these and other SOAs are listed in Table 3.6. The goal of rational drug development is to be able to produce drugs that affect the SOA necessary to mediate the desired effect without affecting an SOA that is not critical to producing the desired effect. Affecting unnecessary SOAs can lead to unnecessary adverse effects and an increased potential for causing pharmacodynamic drug-drug interactions.

Potency Relates to Concentration, Not Dose

There is a frequent misconception that potency refers to the dose of a drug needed to produce an effect. That is wrong. Instead, it refers to the concen-

TABLE 3.4 — RELATIVE POTENCY OF THE ENANTIOMERS OF CITALOPRAM, FLUOXETINE AND THEIR METABOLITES FOR INHIBITING THE UPTAKE PUMPS FOR DIFFERENT BIOGENIC AMINE NEUROTRANSMITTERS

Drug	Inhibitory Concentration, 50% of Maximum Effect (IC50)[1]		
	5HT	NE	DA
Racemic citalopram	1.8	6100	40,000
S-citalopram	1.5	2500	65,000
R-citalopram	250	6900	54,000
S/R ratio* for citalopram = 0.56[2]			
Racemic desmethylcitalopram	14	740	28,000
S-desmethylcitalopram	10	1500	34,000
R-desmethylcitalopram	65	500	25,000
S/R ratio* for desmethylcitalopram = 0.69[2]			

Drug	Kinetic Inhibitory Constant, K_i (nM)[3]		
	5HT	**NE**	**DA**
Racemic fluoxetine	20	1,230	2,880
S-fluoxetine	22	2,040	2,510
R-fluoxetine	35	562	2,820
S/R ratio* for fluoxetine = 2.2[4]			
Racemic norfluoxetine	45	2,400	2,190
S-norfluoxetine	14	4,270	2,750
R-norfluoxetine	309	3,720	2,140
S/R ratio* for norfluoxetine = 2.2[4]			

* *S/R* ratio = ratio of plasma levels of the two enantiomers under steady-state condition when the racemic mixture is being taken.

References: [1]130, [2]242, [3]290, [4]272

TABLE 3.5 — *IN VITRO* SELECTIVITY RATIO* FOR DIFFERENT SSRIS AND SELECTED TCAS			
Drug	Study 1[1]	Study 2[2]	Study 3[3]
Paroxetine	280.0	50.0	64.0
Sertraline	840.0	187.0	45.0
Clomipramine	14.0	6.5	—
Citalopram	3400.0	1015.0	—
Fluvoxamine	160.0	97.0	—
Fluoxetine	54.0	8.0	10.0
Imipramine	0.4	0.3	0.3
Amitriptyline	0.6	0.2	0.2
Desipramine	0.004	0.004	0.003

* (IC50 NE uptake/IC50 5-HT uptake)

References: [1]129, [2]250, [3]34

tration of a drug needed to produce an effect. Two drugs may be able to produce exactly the same effect, but the concentration needed of each drug may be quite different. The drug that requires a lower concentration to achieve the same magnitude of effect is the more potent drug regardless of the dose needed to achieve that concentration.

Although dose is sometimes used as the reference point, it is usually because the concentration has not been measured or the author may not be aware of how misleading a dose comparison can be. The concentration achieved by a given dose of a drug is dependent on the bioavailability and elimination rate of the drug. A drug that has lower bioavailability and/or a faster clearance will require a higher dose to produce the same concentration as a drug which has a greater bioavailability or a slower clearance. The critical issue for the SOA is not what dose is taken, but what concentration is achieved at the SOA.

Table 3.7 illustrates how misleading dose can be, using SSRIs as examples of this basic pharmacological principle. This table shows:

- Usually effective dose of each SSRI
- Usual concentration of each drug at its usually effective dose achieved
- *In vitro* potency for inhibiting the serotonin uptake pump
- *In vivo* degree of serotonin uptake inhibition achieved by each drug at its usually effective, antidepressant dose in man using the platelet as a surrogate for the serotonin neurons since platelets, like serotonin neurons, have a serotonin uptake pump

As can be seen, there is little correlation between the dose of the drug and the plasma concentration achieved. For example, the combined plasma concentration of fluoxetine and its active metabolite,

47

TABLE 3.6 — PHARMACOLOGIC PROPERTIES OF ANTIDEPRESSANTS AND POSSIBLE CLINICAL CONSEQUENCES

Property	Consequences
Blockade of histamine (H-1 and H-2) receptors	Sedation, drowsiness; potentiation of central depressant drugs; weight gain
Blockade of muscarinic acetylcholine receptors	Dry mouth, blurred vision, sinus tachycardia, constipation, urinary retention, memory impairment
Blockade of norepinephrine uptake at nerve endings	Antidepressant efficacy (?); tremors, jitteriness; tachycardia; diaphoresis; blockade of the antihypertensive effects of guanethidine; augmentation of pressor effects of sympathomimetic amines; erectile and ejaculatory dysfunction
Blockade of serotonin uptake at nerve endings	Antidepressant efficacy (?); sexual dysfunction; nausea, vomiting, diarrhea; anorexia; increase or decrease in anxiety (dose-dependent); asthenia (tiredness); insomnia; extrapyramidal side effects; interactions with L-tryptophan, monoamine oxidase inhibitors, fenfluramine, and occasionally lithium
Blockade of serotonin-2 (5-HT2) receptors	Antidepressant efficacy (?), ejaculatory dysfunction, hypotension, alleviation of migraine headaches, decrease in anxiety (?), decrease motor restlessness (?)

Blockade of α_1-adrenergic receptors	Postural hypotension, dizziness which predisposes to falls possibly resulting in broken bones and subdural hematomas, potentiation of antihypertensive drugs
Blockade of α_2-adrenergic receptors	Priapism; blockade of the antihypertensive effects of clonidine, α-methyldopa, guanabenz, guanfacine
Blockade of fast sodium channels	Slow repolarization, delay intracardiac conduction, reduce some arrhythmias at low concentrations, cause arrhythmias, seizures at high concentrations
References: 188, 225, 239	

TABLE 3.7 — RELATIONSHIP BETWEEN DOSE, PLASMA LEVEL, POTENCY AND SEROTONIN (5-HT) UPTAKE

SSRI	Usually Effective Dose (mg/day)*	Plasma Level†	In Vitro Potency IC50‡§	Inhibition of 5-HT Uptake Pump (%)
Citalopram	40	≈ 85 ng/ml (260 nM)[1]	1.8 (14)	≈ 60%[7]
Fluoxetine	20	≈ 200 ng/ml (660 nM)[2]	6.8 (3.8)	≈ 80%[8]
Fluvoxamine	150	≈ 100 ng/ml (300 nM)[3]	3.8	≈ 70%[9]
Paroxetine	20	≈ 40 ng/ml (130 nM)[4]	0.29	≈ 80%[10]
Sertraline	50	≈ 25 ng/ml (65 nM)[5]	0.19 (NA)§	≈ 80%[11]

* Refer to Section 5 for this discussion.
† Plasma level for fluoxetine represents total of fluoxetine plus norfluoxetine given comparable effect of each on 5-HT uptake pump; parent SSRI alone shown for all others. Also, plasma levels are a total of both enantiomers for citalopram and fluoxetine.
‡ Value for parent drug and value for respective major metabolite are in parentheses.
§ Not available from this study. Refer to Table 3.8.

References: [1]31, 93, 146, 179, 197, 242; [2]86, 159, 219, 232; [3]90, 182; [4]21, 122, 166, 167, 252; [5]5, 219, 243; [6]129; [7]31; [8]159; [9]292; [10]170; [11]223

norfluoxetine, is 10 times higher than the concentration of sertraline even though the dose of fluoxetine is 2.5 times less than the dose of sertraline. If the comparison was made on the basis of dose, fluoxetine were erroneously appear to be more potent than sertraline as an inhibitor of serotonin uptake. While the dose of SSRIs does not correlate with their *in vitro* potency, there is a clear correlation between the *in vitro* potency of the drug and the plasma level of each drug needed to produce relatively comparable serotonin uptake inhibition (ie, lower plasma concentrations of the more potent SSRIs [eg, paroxetine, sertraline] are needed in comparison to higher concentrations of the less potent SSRIs [eg, citalopram, fluoxetine, fluvoxamine]).

The results in Table 3.7 are of clinical and research interest. Each SSRI, at the dose found to be its usually effective, minimum dose based on double-blind, placebo-controlled studies, produces approximately 70% to 80% inhibition of the serotonin uptake pump using the platelet as a surrogate marker. This finding is consistent with the concept that the inhibition of this pump is relevant to the antidepressant efficacy of these drugs and suggests that approximately 70% to 80% inhibition of this pump is usually necessary to produce an antidepressant effect. Higher doses of these drugs do not produce a greater antidepressant response on average (ie, a flat dose-response curve for antidepressant efficacy), but do increase the incidence and severity of adverse effects mediated by excessive serotonin uptake inhibition (eg, agitation, loose stools, nausea). (For more details on this issue, refer to Figures 5.1 and 5.2 later in this book.) These two observations, coupled with the results shown in Table 3.7, indicate that inhibition of the serotonin uptake pump by substantially more than 80% produces a greater increase in adverse effects than an increase in antidepressant efficacy and is one reason to avoid the temptation to use a dose higher than the usually effective dose before it has been given an adequate trial (ie, approximately 4 weeks).

Obviously, the results in Table 3.7 pertain to the average patient. A patient who has a rapid clearance of the drug may need a higher than average dose to achieve an effective concentration, whereas a patient who has a slow clearance may do better in terms of the ratio of efficacy-to-adverse effects on a dose lower than usually effective, minimum dose. (For more details on this issue, refer to the *Therapeutic Drug Monitoring* discussion in Section 5.)

The Concept of Selectivity as Related to Effects on Different Neuroreceptors

The goal of development of SSRIs is not only to avoid affecting the norepinephrine and dopamine uptake pumps, but a variety of neuroreceptors (in contrast to the TCAs). Figure 3.3 illustrates how well that goal is accomplished using clomipramine as the reference TCA. Shown in this figure are the binding affinities of 7 different chemical agents (ie, clomipramine and its primary metabolite, desmethylclomipramine, and all SSRIs) for 5 clinically important neuroreceptors as well as the 3 biogenic amine uptake pumps. The X-axis is nanomolar concentration on an algorithmic scale so that each vertical line represents an increase in concentration of ten times the previous one. The further the distance between the drug's affinity for one SOA and the next, the greater its selectivity for affecting that target without affecting the next potential target.

Clomipramine differs from the other tertiary amine TCAs (eg, amitriptyline, doxepin, imipramine) in that its most potent action is on a site believed to mediate

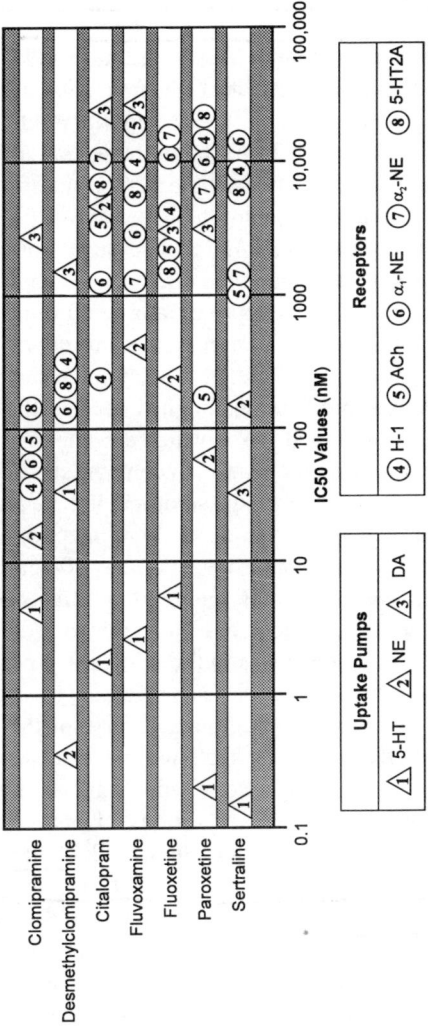

FIGURE 3.3 — *IN VITRO* PROFILE OF ANTIDEPRESSANTS

IC50 Values (nM)

| Uptake Pumps |
| △ 5-HT △ NE △ DA |

| Receptors |
| ④ H-1 ⑤ ACh ⑥ α₁-NE ⑦ α₂-NE ⑧ 5-HT2A |

efficacy in major depression and also obsessive-compulsive disorders (ie, the serotonin uptake pump). In contrast, the other tertiary amine TCAs block the histamine receptor as their most potent action, which is why their most potent effect is sedation and why they can potentiate the effect of other sedative agents, including alcohol.[76,123,155,188,211,251] Clomipramine, like the other tertiary amine TCAs, has little separation between potency for effects on multiple SOAs such as the norepinephrine uptake pump, the histamine-1, α-1 adrenergic, acetylcholine, 5-HT2A neuroreceptors and the dopamine uptake pump (Figure 3.3). The widest gap for clomipramine is approximately 300 times for the inhibition of the serotonin versus the dopamine uptake pump. That difference is such that clomipramine is unlikely to produce meaningful effects on the dopamine uptake pump at doses which substantially inhibit the serotonin uptake pump. In contrast, the difference between its affinity for the serotonin uptake pump and the other neural SOAs (eg, the norepinephrine uptake pump and various neuroreceptors) is 10-fold or less. That difference is small enough that effects on these sites may occur under clinically relevant conditions and thus can contribute to the clinical pharmacology of the drug. If clinical effects mediated by the drug's action on these sites are unnecessary for the desired clinical effects, these effects will be termed "side-effects" and may range from being a nuisance to treatment-limiting problems to serious adverse effects.

Although not shown in Figure 3.3, clomipramine, like the other TCAs, is also capable of inhibiting fast sodium channels.[57] The potency of the drug for this action is such that it occurs to a clinically meaningful extent in the healthy individual only at concentrations above its therapeutic range for antidepressant efficacy and the probable reason for its dose- and, hence, concentration-dependent seizure risk and cardiac arrhythmia risk.[59] However, concentrations can occur in individuals who take an overdose of the drug or who are slow metabolizers and develop high concentrations on what are usually therapeutic doses.[221,225] Slow metabolizers are typically deficient in the cytochrome P450 enzyme, CYP 2D6, either because of genetics or because they are on a concomitant drug that substantially inhibits this enzyme (eg, fluoxetine or paroxetine).[45,213]

3

Inhibition of fast sodium channels produces stabilization of electrically excitable membranes and clinically results in the potentially life-threatening adverse effects that TCAs can have on the heart (eg, conduction disturbances) and the brain (eg, seizures).[33,222,225] Thus, effects of TCAs on this SOA cause their narrow therapeutic index.

Figure 3.3 illustrates another complicating feature of the pharmacology of clomipramine and the other tertiary amine TCAs. They are demethylated in the body to secondary amine TCAs which have a pharmacological profile different from that of the parent drug. In the case of clomipramine, this metabolite is desmethylclomipramine. Its binding affinity for the same SOAs is shown in Figure 3.3 in the bar below that for the parent drug. As can be seen, this metabolite, like all secondary amine TCAs, is considerably more potent than the parent drug as an inhibitor of the norepinephrine uptake pump and less potent as an inhibitor of the serotonin uptake pump.[34] The conversion of clomipramine to desmethylclomipramine is mediated by at least two CYP enzymes, CYP 1A2 and 3A3/4,[43,44] and possibly 2C19.[168] Activity of these 2 enzymes can vary substantially among individuals and even within the same person because these enzymes can be induced and inhibited by environmental factors, including concomitant medications taken by the individual (discussed further in Sections 7 and 8).

If inhibition of the serotonin uptake pump is critical to the desired clinical effect of clomipramine (eg, efficacy in some forms of major depression and in obsessive-compulsive disorder), then a patient may fail to respond because s/he develops higher levels of the metabolite as opposed to the parent drug. Conceivably, a patient who had responded might lose efficacy if exposed to an environmental agent capable of inducing CYP 1A2 or 3A3/4 after being stabilized on what had previously been an optimal dose of clomipramine. While the physician can increase the dose of clomipramine sufficiently to achieve high enough levels of the parent drug to produce the necessary inhibition of the serotonin uptake pump, the dose may have to be so high that effects of the metabolite on other SOAs can become clinically meaningful, causing nuisance and/or serious adverse effects. Thus, Figure 3.3 illustrates the potential problems inherent in having an active metabolite with a pharmacological profile which is meaningfully different from the parent compound.

Figure 3.3 also shows the binding affinities for all of the SSRIs. The most potent action of each SSRI is the inhibition of the serotonin uptake pump. Each has a substantially higher affinity for this SOA than for any other site shown. Stated in another way, the SSRIs as a group show a clinically meaningful separation or selectivity for the serotonin uptake pump versus any of the other SOAs shown in Figure 3.3.

However, Figure 3.3 does not show the affinity of these drugs for various CYP enzymes. In the case of these enzymes, some of the SSRIs produce meaningful effects at the same concentration that they affect the serotonin uptake pump and, thus, do not show "selectivity" in terms of distinguishing between the serotonin uptake pump and such CYP enzymes; but instead, they can produce effects on both of these sites under clinically relevant conditions (discussed further in Sections 7 and 8).

What About the Effects of SSRI Metabolites?

Given the discussion of clomipramine and desmethylclomipramine, it is important to know whether SSRIs have active metabolites with a substantially different pharmacological profile than the parent drug. Table 3.8 shows the results of two *in vitro* studies examining the effects of some of the SSRIs and their primary metabolites. The results for clomipramine and desmethylclomipramine, illustrated in Figure 3.3, are shown for comparison purposes. There are two entries for fluoxetine and norfluoxetine because they were examined in both *in vitro* studies.

As can be seen in Table 3.8, the metabolites of citalopram, fluoxetine and sertraline have the same rank order of binding affinity for these various SOAs as their respective parent SSRI. Metabolites of fluvoxamine and paroxetine were not available for testing in these studies, but they are reported to not have metabolites with clinically meaningful affinity for any of these SOAs.[141,198]

The metabolites of citalopram and sertraline are more than 10 times less potent than the parent drug for inhibiting the serotonin uptake pump (Table 3.8). In the case of sertraline, its metabolite is 25 times less potent than the parent drug. Since this metabolite occurs in concentrations only 1.5 times higher than the parent drug under clinically relevant conditions,[219] this metabolite will be expected to contribute negligibly (ie, approximately 6%) to the overall clinical pharmacology of this drug mediated by inhibition of this SOA.

The reverse is true for fluoxetine. In some *in vitro* studies, its primary metabolite, norfluoxetine, has been found to be somewhat more potent than the parent drug at inhibiting the serotonin uptake pump (Table 3.8). Moreover, norfluoxetine levels can be twice the levels

TABLE 3.8 — EFFECT OF UPTAKE INHIBITORS AND THEIR METABOLITES *IN VITRO*

	5-HT uptake	NA uptake	DA uptake	D-2	5-HT2	α_1	H-1	ACh
Clomipramine[1]	1.5	21.0	4,300	430	120	60	54	67
Desmethylclomipramine[1]	40.0	0.45	2,100	1,200	340	190	450	92
Citalopram[1]	1.8	6,100.0	40,000	33,000	9,200	1,600	350	5,600
Desmethylcitalopram[1]	14.0	740.0	28,000	53,000	19,000	1,500	1,700	14,000
Didesmethylcitalopram[1]	22.0	1,400.0	11,000	24,000	16,000	3,400	11,000	23,000
Fluoxetine[1]	6.8	370.0	5,000	32,000	2,600	14,000	3,200	3,100
Norfluoxetine[1]	3.8	580.0	4,300	13,000	2,500	15,000	11,000	3,400
Fluoxetine[2]	14.0	143.0	3,050	12,000	280	3,800	5,400	590
Norfluoxetine[2]	25.0	416.0	1,100	16,000	600	3,900	11,000	810
Sertraline[2]	3.4	220.0	260	11,000	9,900	380	24,000	630
Desmethylsertraline[2]	76.0	420.0	440	11,000	4,800	1,200	9,000	1,430

Note the effects of fluoxetine and norfluoxetine were measured in two different sets of studies. Data from reference 129 are in terms of inhibition concentration, 50% maximum effect (IC50), whereas data from references 34 and 66 are in terms of kinetic inhibition constant (K_i) for the uptake pumps and kinetic dissociation constant (K_d) for the receptors.

References: [1]129, [2]34, 66

of the parent drug and persist for a substantially longer interval after discontinuation due to its slower clearance (ie, longer half-life).[142,219,232] Given its affinity for the serotonin pump and its higher, longer-lived levels, norfluoxetine is an important metabolite with regard to clinical effects mediated by the inhibition of the serotonin uptake pump.

There is an important caveat to this discussion. When the statement is made that a drug does not have an "active metabolite," several questions should be asked:

- How well has the metabolism of the drug been clarified?
- Can there be clinically meaningful metabolites that have not been studied or have not yet been identified?
- What does "active" mean or, in other words, what activity has been studied?

With the exception of fluoxetine, none of the SSRIs have metabolites with clinically relevant effects on any of the neural sites shown in Table 3.8. However, every SSRI that has been studied has metabolites with approximately the same activity as the parent drug for the inhibition of specific CYP enzymes (for details, see Table 8.7). Hence, these metabolites are "active" with regard to inhibiting these enzymes and contributing to the effects mediated by this action (eg, the slowing of the clearance of drugs metabolized by these specific enzymes). The magnitude of the contribution by the metabolite relative to the parent drug is a function of their relative potency for the specific mechanism of action (MOA) of interest and their relative concentrations at the relevant SOA under clinically relevant dosing conditions. For example, norfluoxetine is almost 10 times more potent than the parent drug at inhibiting the CYP enzyme, 3A3/4 (Table 8.7).

TABLE 3.9 — EFFECT OF METABOLISM ON THE CENTRAL MOA AND HALF-LIVES OF SOME SSRIS

Drug	5-HT uptake*[1]	NE uptake[1]	Half-lives*[2]	Consequence
Clomipramine	1.5	2.1	19 to 37 hrs[2]	Loss of selectivity
Desmethylclomipramine	40.0	0.45	54 to 77 hrs[2]	
Fluoxetine	6.8	370.0	2 to 4 days[2,3]	Increased duration of action
Norfluoxetine	3.8	580.0	7 to 15 days[2,3]	
Citalopram	1.8	6100.0	1.5 days[4]	No change in selectivity or duration of action; no clinically active metabolites in terms of serotonin uptake inhibition[†]
Fluvoxamine	3.8	620.0	0.5 to 1 day[5]	
Paroxetine	0.29	81.0	1 day (at 20 mg/d)[2]	
Sertraline	0.19	160.0	1 day[2]	

* Half-live is a major determinant of the duration of action of a drug.

† Metabolites of citalopram and sertraline are substantially weaker inhibitors of serotonin uptake than the parent drug. These metabolites also occur in concentrations either about the same as the parent drug or less. Hence, they do not contribute in a meaningful way to the effect of the drug via this mechanism of action. However, the metabolites of several SSRIs are as potent or more potent as the parent drug at inhibiting specific CYP enzymes and thus contribute to this effect (Table 8.7).

References: [1]129, [2]213, [3]108, [4]173, [5]73

Clinical Relevance of Active Metabolites

The clinical implications of the differential effects of the metabolites of clomipramine and the SSRIs on neural SOAs are summarized in Table 3.9. In the case of clomipramine, its metabolite can cause a loss of selectivity in terms of effects mediated by the inhibition of the serotonin versus the norepinephrine uptake pump. In the case of fluoxetine, its primary metabolite has the same pharmacological profile as the parent drug. In fact, norfluoxetine, relative to fluoxetine:

- Is a comparable or even more potent inhibitor of the serotonin uptake pump and CYP 2D6 (Table 8.7)
- Is a more potent inhibitor of CYP 3A3/4 (Table 8.7)
- Is generally present at higher levels[142,219,232]
- Persists for a substantially longer period of time after fluoxetine administration has been stopped[112,200,219]

For these reasons, this metabolite is clinically important in terms of increasing the magnitude and the duration of clinical effects mediated by the inhibition of the serotonin uptake pump and for effects (eg, pharmacokinetic drug interactions) mediated by the inhibition of one or more CYP enzymes.

With regard to the other SSRIs, they do not have metabolites with sufficient activity at any known neural SOAs to alter or contribute to the magnitude or duration of any psychiatric effects produced by the parent drug. However, the primary metabolites of citalopram, paroxetine and sertraline, like fluoxetine, have similar potency to their respective parent drug in terms of the effects on specific CYP enzymes (for details, see Section 8). The primary metabolites of fluvoxamine have not been adequately studied to comment about this SSRI in this respect.

Conclusion

Understanding the rational development strategy that have been used to produce the SSRIs lays the foundation for understanding their basic neuropharmacology and why it differs from TCAs. This knowledge also explains why the SSRIs are alike in so many ways and also why the differences in their pharmacokinetics and effects on CYP enzymes have become distinguishing characteristics among these drugs.

4

How SSRIs as a Group
Differ From TCAs

The goal behind the rational development of selective serotonin reuptake inhibitors (SSRIs) is to:
- Either maintain or ideally enhance antidepressant efficacy
- Increase the therapeutic index (ie, the safety margin between the effective versus the toxic dose)
- Improve the tolerability profile
- Reduce the risk of pharmacodynamically mediated drug-drug interactions

This development plan has succeeded relative to tricyclic antidepressants (TCAs). Hence, SSRIs, for many physicians, have replaced TCAs as antidepressants of first choice in the treatment of patients with major depression. They also have increased the likelihood that a patient with symptoms of major depression will receive a trial of an antidepressant at an optimal dose. The reason for the increased likelihood of a trial of antidepressant is that physicians are more comfortable giving an empirical trial of SSRIs than a trial of TCAs due to their wider safety margin and better tolerability. The likelihood that an optimal dose will be used is that there is no need to titrate the dose of SSRIs for most patients. The starting dose is the optimal for most patients. Dose increases, in general, serve little purpose.

The differences in the clinical pharmacology of TCAs versus SSRIs will be reviewed in this chapter in terms of the STEPS analysis developed by the author (Table 4.1).

TABLE 4.1 — STEPS: FACTORS TO BE CONSIDERED WHEN SELECTING A MEDICATION FOR A PATIENT

- **S**afety
  - Acute therapeutic index
  - Long-term safety
  - Risk of drug-drug interactions:
    - Pharmacodynamically mediated
    - Pharmacokinetically mediated
- **T**olerability
  - Acute
  - Long-term
- **E**fficacy
  - Overall response rate
  - Unique spectrum of activity in subpopulations
  - Rate of onset
  - Maintenance
  - Prophylactic
- **P**ayment (ie, cost-effectiveness)
- **S**implicity
  - Drug administration schedule
  - Ease of optimal dosing
  - Need for specific clinical or laboratory monitoring before or during treatment

References: 49, 210

Safety

Table 4.2 summarizes the clinically meaningful differences between TCAs and SSRIs in terms of safety and tolerability. Due to the fact that SSRIs do not inhibit fast sodium channels, there is essentially no risk of lethality, even with a substantial overdose of these medications. In contrast, overdoses of a TCA of as little as 5 times the daily dose can be lethal.[225] This issue is important because of the delay between starting an antidepressant of any class and achieving a meaningful improvement in the depressive syndrome.

TABLE 4.2 — SAFETY AND TOLERABILITY OF TCAS VERSUS SSRIS

Consideration	TCAs	SSRIs
Safety		
Overdose lethality risk	high	low
Alcohol potentiation	high	low
Tolerability		
Anticholingeric adverse events	high	low
Antihistamine adverse events	high	low
Anti-α_1 adrenergic adverse events	high	low
Serotonin adverse events	low	high

The risk of a suicide attempt is a serious concern during this delayed onset interval. For many years, TCAs have been a leading cause of death due to drug overdose because of their serious toxicity profile, coupled with the fact that they are given to patients at risk for making serious suicide attempts.[52,97,165] Because SSRIs avoid this problem, the prognosis of patients suffering from this condition has significantly improved.

It used to be axiomatic to warn patients about the dangers of drinking alcohol while taking antidepressants. While it is still wise to advise patients against drinking alcohol when clinically depressed, the reason is no longer because the antidepressant will necessarily cause serious potentiation of the central nervous system (CNS) depressant effects of alcohol and other CNS depressants such as benzodiazepines. Such potentiation occurs when TCAs and alcohol are taken together due to the antihistaminic effects of TCAs, particularly tertiary amine TCAs. Since SSRIs have been designed to avoid blocking the histamine receptor, they do not pharmacodynamically potentiate the effect of alcohol or other CNS depressants.[76,123,155,251] Instead, they either do nothing or may mildly antagonize the depressant effects of alcohol.[76,123,155,251] This change is just one example of the reduced risk of serious pharmacodynamic drug interactions due to the more focused pharmacology of SSRIs. Parenthetically, fluvoxamine and fluoxetine can pharmacokinetically potentiate the effects of 2-keto and triazolo benzodiazepines, such as diazepam and alprazolam respectively, by inhibiting the cytochrome P450 (CYP) enzymes responsible for their clearance (see Section 8).

The avoidance of pharmacodynamically mediated drug-drug interactions is important because of the length of time that patients may be on antidepressants to prevent relapse or recurrence of depressive illness. As discussed in Section 8, antidepressants are frequently used in combination with other drugs for a variety of reasons:

- Concomitant medical illness
- Augmentation strategies
- The addition of another drug to reduce a nuisance adverse effect (eg, cisapride to treat nausea which can occur early in SSRI treatment)

In addition, patients may drink alcohol socially while taking an antidepressant and then try to drive home. Alternatively, they may take "over-the-counter" (OTC) preparations and have an interaction (ie, taking an OTC drug that has sedative properties). If they are taking a tertiary amine TCA and drink alcohol or take such an OTC product, they may experience serious potentiation of sedative effects that may be dangerous, particularly if they are in a situation where they need to be mentally alert with good reaction time and coordination.

Due to the multiple pharmacodynamic effects of TCAs, there are multiple ways that they can interact with other types of drugs beyond simply the potentiation of CNS depressants. Since TCAs block α_1-adrenergic receptors, they lower peripheral resistance.[103] If the patient is also taking other medications that lower blood pressure (eg, diuretics, ß-blockers), they may experience a marked potentiation of the orthostatic hypotension that can occur with drugs that block α_1-adrenergic receptors, that can have serious consequences in terms of falls and resultant trauma, particularly in the elderly.[236] Since SSRIs have been also designed to avoid blocking the α_1-adrenergic receptor, they do not potentiate the effects of concomitantly prescribed antihypertensive medications, in contrast to TCAs. This is another example of the reduced risk of pharmacodynamically mediated drug interactions as a result of the more focused pharmacology of SSRIs.

Since TCAs block the muscarinic acetylcholine receptor, they can have additive effects with other drugs that also block this receptor or which affect gastrointestinal tract motility through other actions. Since TCAs inhibit fast sodium channels, they can potentiate the effects of other drugs which affect intracardiac conduction. Such drugs include a variety of antiarrhythmics, calcium channel blockers, and β-blockers. SSRIs, because of their more focused pharmacology, have a much more limited range of pharmacodynamically mediated drug-drug interactions than do TCAs.

Tolerability

Another important difference between SSRIs and TCAs is a better overall tolerability profile in terms of a lower incidence of both nuisance and serious adverse effects. SSRIs affect fewer sites of action (SOAs) and hence cause fewer types of adverse effects. Table 4.3 shows the relative incidence of adverse effects on imipramine as a representative TCA. Imipramine was chosen because it has historically been and still is one of the most commonly used TCAs. Table 5.2 shows the relative incidence of the same adverse effects on 4 of the 5 SSRIs. A comparison of these 2 tables reveals that imipramine in comparison to the SSRIs is

TABLE 4.3 — PLACEBO-ADJUSTED INCIDENCE RATE (%) OF FREQUENT ADVERSE EFFECTS ON IMIPRAMINE*

Headache	− 8.7
Nervousness	3.6
Tremors	10.0
Insomnia	0.4
Drowsiness	12.0
Fatigue	7.6
Anorexia	—
Dizziness	22.7
Vision disturbance	5.4
Palpitations	—
Respiration	− 2.3
Nausea	1.3
Dyspepsia	—
Diarrhea	− 2.7
Dry mouth	47.1
Constipation	17.4
Frequent micturition	—
Urinary retention	4.0
Sweating	11.2

* n = 367, placebo = 672

Placebo-adjusted = incidence on drug minus incidence on parallel, placebo group in a double-blind, randomly assigned clinical trial.

Data from reference: 211

associated with a considerably higher incidence of adverse effects mediated by the blockade of specific neuroreceptors such as muscarinic acetylcholine receptors (eg, dry mouth, constipation) and α_1-adrenergic receptors (eg, dizziness). In contrast, SSRIs as a group have a higher incidence of adverse effects mediated by the indirect potentiation of serotonin via the inhibition of its uptake pump (eg, nausea). Figure 4.1 provides a visual representation of the same phenomena using amitriptyline as another representative tertiary amine TCA and sertraline as a representative SSRI.

While these adverse effects are less dramatic than the potentially life-threatening toxicity problems that can occur while taking TCAs, they can have serious consequences. The orthostatic hypotension that can occur on TCAs may cause falls with resultant trauma.[236] The chronic anticholinergic effects can lead the patient to discontinue treatment during the maintenance phase of treatment and thus increase the risk of relapse. In clinical studies, the discontinuation of tertiary amine TCAs such as imipramine can be 3 times higher than the discontinuation rate on an SSRI (eg, 22% versus 7% respectively).[211]

Efficacy

While rational drug development reduces the risk of safety and tolerability problems with SSRIs versus TCAs, it does not reduce the relative antidepressant efficacy of the SSRIs. As a group, they are as effective as TCAs in the treatment of outpatients with major depression. This conclusion is supported by a meta-analysis of the double-blind clinical trials of TCAs and SSRIs versus placebo and the double-blind trials directly comparing the antidepressant efficacy of SSRIs and TCAs (Table 4.4). In this table, efficacy is presented as response rate on each treatment after a 6-week treatment trial. A responder is defined as a patient who experienced at least a 50% reduction in the depressive symptomatology as assessed by a standard-

FIGURE 4.1 — COMPARATIVE INCIDENCE OF SIDE EFFECTS BETWEEN AMITRIPTYLINE AND SERTRALINE

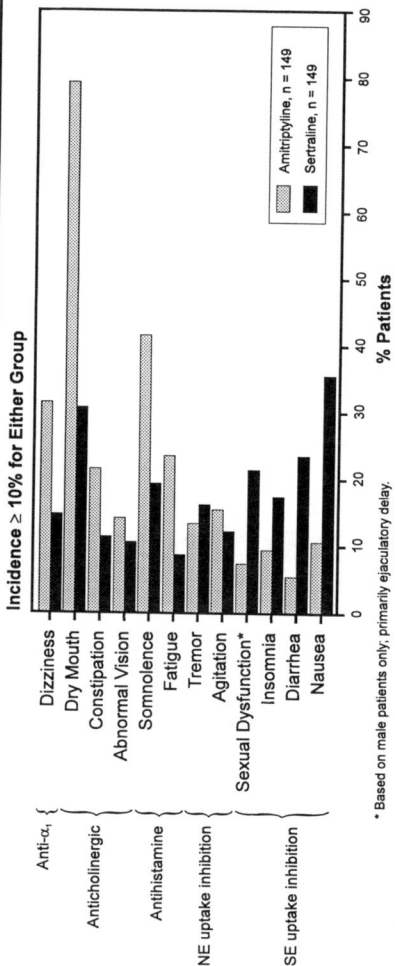

Incidence ≥ 10% for Either Group

Anti-α₁: Dizziness

Anticholinergic: Dry Mouth, Constipation, Abnormal Vision

Antihistamine: Somnolence, Fatigue

NE uptake inhibition: Tremor, Agitation

SE uptake inhibition: Sexual Dysfunction*, Insomnia, Diarrhea, Nausea

% Patients

Amitriptyline, n = 149
Sertraline, n = 149

* Based on male patients only; primarily ejaculatory delay.

Treatment-emergent side effects (all causalities) in double-blind, placebo-controlled, outpatient trial.

Reference: 237

TABLE 4.4 — RESPONSE RATES IN PATIENTS WITH MAJOR DEPRESSIVE DISORDER BY META-ANALYSIS

TCAs and SSRIs (*as a class*) vs. Placebo	Drug	Placebo	Difference	n	*p* value
TCAs	62.8%	35.9%	26.9%	5159	$< 10^{-40}$
SSRIs	66.5%	38.1%	28.4%	2216	$< 10^{-30}$
	SSRI	TCA	Difference	n	*p* value
TCAs vs. SSRIs	77.2	76.9	0.3%	850	NS

NS = Not significant

From reference: 135

ized assessment instrument, such as the Hamilton Depression Rating Scale (HDRS).

The conclusion that TCAs and SSRIs have comparable antidepressant efficacy in this group of patients is based on the fact that they both produce overall response rates of 60% to 65% and that these rates are comparably superior to those achieved in a double-blind, parallel, placebo-treated, control group. Both the SSRIs and the TCAs produce a 25% to 30% higher response rate than placebo. This difference between drug and placebo is also statistically superior to a comparable degree.

Nonetheless, these results do not necessarily mean that exactly the same patients respond to SSRIs and TCAs. Some investigators have suggested that TCAs may work better in patients who are hospitalized for major depression.[69,70,244] That opinion is based on a few double-blind, active, controlled studies. However, this issue remains controversial and is not presently resolved. There are also studies showing that up to 50% patients who fail to respond to desipramine or a similar TCA will respond to an SSRI and vice versa.[1,2,81,124,164,190,191] That finding further suggests that the spectrum of antidepressant activity by these 2 classes of drugs is not identical. However, considerable work needs to be done to confirm or reject these hypotheses. Nonetheless, current data do suggest that it is clinically reasonable to give a patient who has failed on an SSRI a trial of a TCA or related drug as well as vice versa.

Payment

This topic is clearly important and is part of the STEPS analysis.[49] However, a full discussion is beyond the scope of this book, given its focus on clinical pharmacology. Nonetheless, the clinical pharmacology of SSRIs versus TCAs must be considered when analyzing the issue of payment or cost-effectiveness of these different classes of antidepressants. The acquisition cost of SSRIs is higher than that of TCAs but that is only one part of the cost-effectiveness equation. To be meaningful, a cost-effectiveness analysis must be much more comprehensive and consider such factors as:

- The cost of administering the treatment
  - Number of physician visits
  - Ancillary tests that are needed to monitor the treatment
- The cost of treating potential adverse outcomes that may range from nuisance side effects to serious toxicity such as can occur with an overdose of a TCA
- The cost of an adverse outcome due to an adverse drug-drug interaction
- The cost of effective treatment must be balanced against the cost of not effectively treating the illness (eg, loss productivity), including increased relapse rates in patients who discontinue treatment before the drug has a chance to work or who relapse because of discontinuing treatment too early because of intolerable side effects

Simplicity

Simplicity refers to how easy it is for the physician to prescribe the optimal dose and for the patient to take it. One advantage shared by both TCAs and SSRIs is that they can generally be taken once a day and be effective. Other than this shared feature, optimal dosing with TCAs is often more problematic than with SSRIs.

Traditionally, treatment with TCAs is begun at what is usually a subtherapeutic dose and gradually titrated upward to an effective antidepressant dose.

This approach is taken so that the patient can develop some tolerance to the adverse effects caused by these drugs due to their ability to block specific neuro-receptors as discussed earlier in this section. In contrast, SSRIs as a class can usually be started at the effective dose from the beginning. As discussed in the next section, there is generally no need to titrate the dose of the SSRIs upward in most patients.

With TCAs, the physician can use therapeutic drug monitoring (TDM) to ensure that the patient is achieving plasma drug concentration within a range associated with the optimal antidepressant response with the minimum risk of adverse effects in most patients.[221] This is an advantage from a clinical pharmacology perspective, but is often viewed as a cumbersome disadvantage from a clinical practice standpoint. As discussed in the next section, TDM can also be used with SSRIs for the same purpose, although it is rarely done.

The difference between TCAs and SSRIs with regard to TDM is that it is a standard of care issue with TCAs, but not with SSRIs, due to the difference in their therapeutic indexes (ie, the difference between a dose that is therapeutic and one that is toxic). Patients who are slow metabolizers of TCAs can develop potentially toxic concentrations on conventional antidepressant doses of these medications because of the multiple SOAs affected by TCAs over their clinically relevant pharmacological range. If the patient slowly clears these drugs either due to a genetically- or environmentally-induced deficiency in the cytochrome P450 enzymes responsible for their biotransformation and eventual elimination, they can develop concentrations that affect fast sodium channels and, hence, delay intracardiac conduction. Sufficient slowing can lead to conduction delays and set the stage for potentially life-threatening cardiac arrhythmias even though the patient is taking what is normally a therapeutic dose. The avoidance of potentially toxic concentrations is the primary reason for using TDM with TCAs.[221]

74

5 How SSRIs as a Group Are Similar

The rational drug discovery used to produce the selective serotonin reuptake inhibitors (SSRIs) explains why they are similar as a class in so many ways (Table 5.1) as well as why they differ as a class from tricyclic antidepressants (TCAs). As in the preceding chapter, a summary of the similarities among the SSRIs using the STEPS approach will be given rather than an exhaustive review.

Ideally, this chapter would be based on data from studies in which patients were randomly assigned to one of several treatment arms: one for each SSRI at

---

TABLE 5.1 — COMMON FEATURES OF SSRIS WITH REGARD TO THE TREATMENT OF MAJOR DEPRESSION

- Flat-dose antidepressant-response curve
- Equivalent antidepressant efficacy at their usually effective, therapeutic dose: 40 mg/d for citalopram, 20 mg/d for fluoxetine and paroxetine, and 50 mg/d for sertraline*
- Similar efficacy when used on maintenance basis to prevent relapses
- Usually effective, minimum dose for each SSRI produces approximately 60% to 80% inhibition of serotonin uptake
- Benign adverse effect profile compared to TCAs

* Comparable data from fixed-dose studies not available for fluvoxamine.

---

their respective, comparable antidepressant doses and one for a placebo. Ideally, these studies would contain an adequate number of patients randomly assigned to each of these discrete treatment arms to determine whether there are meaningful differences with regard to safety, tolerability and efficacy. Since there are 5 SSRIs, such studies would have at a minimum 6 treatment groups (ie, each SSRI and the placebo arm). Most researchers would probably not want to gamble on doing such a study with only 1 dose per drug because of the criticism that the dose chosen for a given SSRI was not the truly comparable dose for that drug and thus biased the study outcome relative to that drug. Instead, they would have more than 1 dose arm for each SSRI. However, each dose added per drug would multiply the number of groups needed for the study and thus its size and complexity. To adequately power these studies to test for expected differences between these different drugs would require hundreds of patients per group. Given these considerations, it should not be surprising that such studies do not exist. Moreover, such studies will almost undoubtably never be done for quite practical reasons of cost and logistics.

Since the ideal data does not exist for the purposes of this book, the next best approach is taken by relying on summary data from comparable studies of rigorous design. To be included, the data has to come from double-blind, placebo-controlled, adequately powered studies. The presence of a placebo group permits comparisons to be drawn across the studies by comparing the drugs on the basis of placebo-adjusted differences in such outcome variables as adverse effects and efficacy. In some instances, comparable data has not been published for all of the SSRIs and, therefore, some SSRIs cannot be included in the analysis. Those instances are pointed out in the text.

Safety

There are multiple facets to this broad heading, including:

- Therapeutic index
- Long-term safety
- Risk of pharmacodynamically and pharmacokinetically mediated drug-drug interactions

The available data indicate that the SSRIs as a group are remarkably similar in all of these ways with the exception of pharmacokinetically mediated drug-drug interactions. Given the complexity of that topic and the fact that it is a major distinguishing characteristic of these otherwise quite similar drugs, it is discussed at length in Sections 7 and 8.

Since all SSRIs have been designed to avoid affecting fast sodium channels in contrast to TCAs, they all have a wide therapeutic index (ie, the gap between the effective dose and a potentially toxic dose). They do not affect intracardiac conduction.[36,100,165] Patients have survived overdoses of each of the SSRIs that were many times their usually effective antidepressant doses without serious toxicity including:

- No arrhythmias
- No disturbance of blood pressure
- No seizures
- No coma
- No respiratory depression

All of these adverse effects do occur with overdose of TCAs as little as 5 times their therapeutic doses.[225] In most instances of an overdose of only an SSRI, there is no need for medical intervention beyond observation and addressing the reasons for the overdose.[36,100,165]

Drug-drug interactions, whether pharmacodynamically or pharmacokinetically mediated, are a safety issue with any drug since polypharmacy is a common clinical practice particularly in the most fragile patients (ie, the elderly and those with multiple medical illnesses). As mentioned above, pharmacokinetically mediated drug-drug interactions with SSRIs will be the subject of a latter section; however, this phenomenon will be briefly mentioned here since there is overdose risk with these drugs when they are taken in combination with other drugs.

Overdoses in the form of a suicide attempt are typically done with more than one drug.[36,100,165] SSRI-induced inhibition of a specific cytochrome P450 (CYP) enzyme can affect the toxicity resulting from such an overdose in two ways due to inhibition of the CYP enzyme which mediates the metabolism of the concomitant drug. If the concomitantly ingested drug normally has extensive first pass metabolism dependent on that enzyme, then SSRI-induced inhibition of that enzyme should increase the bioavailability of the other drug and thus increase the toxicity of the overdose. The inhibition of the enzyme should also delay the clearance of the other drugs and thus increase the duration of their toxicity. An increased duration will involve longer care and potentially an increased risk of time-dependent sequelae such as intercurrent infection in an overdose patient with compromised ventilation due to respiratory depression. One example would is an overdose involving a TCA and an SSRI that is capable of causing substantial inhibition of the metabolism of TCAs (eg, fluoxetine- or paroxetine-induced inhibition of CYP 2D6) (refer to Section 8 for details).

There can be many other examples involving overdoses with a wide range of drugs from benzodiazepines to cardiovascular drugs to narcotics. This scenario is based on the known pharmacology of these drugs and pharmacokinetic principles, but to date there are no studies which have tested whether this scenario meaningfully affects clinical outcome in such multiple drug overdoses.

A reduced risk of pharmacodynamically mediated drug-drug interactions is a class advantage of SSRIs over TCAs as discussed in Section 4. Nonetheless, SSRIs can have pharmacodynamically mediated adverse drug-drug interactions, primarily with drugs that also affect serotonin mechanisms of actions (MOAs). Such interactions are a class issue common to all of the SSRIs and a direct result of the MOA they were designed to share (ie, the inhibition of serotonin uptake). The most serious of these adverse interactions is the central serotonin syndrome that can occur when monoamine oxidase inhibitors (MAOIs) are combined with SSRIs.[266] Minor variants of this syndrome in terms of the number of symptoms, their severity, and their duration can occur when a variety of serotonin active drugs (eg, lithium, busiprone) are added to SSRIs or MAOIs.

This pharmacodynamically mediated drug interaction results from the combined indirect serotonin agonism caused by both the inhibition of serotonin degradation produced by the MAOI and the inhibition of serotonin uptake produced by the SSRI. Together, these two actions can create a potentially catastrophic dysregulation of a variety of basic brainstem mechanisms, regulated by the central serotonin neural system and produce a syndrome consisting of:

- Hyperthermia
- Diaphoresis
- Gastrointestinal distress
- Mental status changes
- Myoclonus[266]

The central serotonin syndrome produced by the combined use of SSRIs and MAOIs is particularly dangerous because of its severity and duration due to the persistent action of MAOIs. The duration may also be increased the longer the half-life of the SSRI. In severe cases, this interaction can be fatal.

To avoid this interaction, SSRIs should not be started until 2 weeks after the discontinuation of MAOIs to allow for replenishment of MAO activity. Similarly, MAOIs should not be started until there has been virtual full washout of the SSRIs, which takes 2 weeks for all of the SSRIs except fluoxetine. A minimum of 5 weeks is recommended for fluoxetine if the daily dose was 20 mg/day, and longer if the daily dose was higher, due to the nonlinear pharmacokinetics of fluoxetine (see Section 6).

Tolerability

While the SSRIs as a class differ from the TCAs in terms of avoiding a number of adverse effects that are mediated by the blockade of histamine, acetylcholine, and α_1-adrenergic receptors, as well as fast sodium channels, all SSRIs as a class produce adverse effects that are the result of the MOA they are designed to share (ie, indirect serotonin agonism by inhibiting the serotonin uptake pump). mechanism of action

The adverse effects produced by a drug can be determined in several ways.[211] The most common is by determining what adverse complaints or physiological effects are seen to a statistically significant greater degree in the drug-treated group versus a parallel placebo-treated group. Table 5.2 presents the data on this issue for 4 of the SSRIs: fluvoxamine, fluoxetine, paroxetine and sertraline. The data in this table is from the double-blind, placebo-controlled clinical trial databases with these 4 SSRIs. The presence of the placebo control allowed for a comparison of the placebo-adjusted rates of specific adverse effects for these 4 SSRIs (ie, the incidence rate of each specific SSRI minus the incidence rate that occurred on its parallel, double-blind, placebo control). The reader who is interested in a further discussion of this approach is referred to a recent paper on this subject.[211] Unfortunately, comparable data for citalopram is not available for this analysis. Hence, comparative statements about the rate of specific adverse effects cannot be made about citalopram. Nevertheless, citalopram has been reported to produce the same type of adverse effects now known to be caused by serotonin uptake inhibition.[173]

As can be readily seen in Table 5.2, there are only modest differences in the incidence rates for various adverse effects for these different SSRIs consistent with how these drugs are developed. Since data in this table are from the clinical trials databases with these drugs, it represents the average incidence on the various doses of that SSRI used in its clinical trials. The incidence and severity of many of these adverse effects are dose-dependent as seen in Figure 5.1, which shows the discontinuation rate due to adverse effects as a function of dose for the 3 SSRIs which have published fixed-dose studies.

Given the dose-dependent nature of many of SSRI-mediated adverse effects, a specific SSRI can be at a disadvantage in Figures 5.1 and 5.2 and Table 5.3 if the doses used predominantly in its clinical trials development were higher than its usually effective, therapeutic dose while the other SSRIs were dosed closer to their usually effective dose. In fact, the use of higher than necessary doses was the case for virtually all of the SSRIs, particularly in the early phases of their clinical trials. The reason is that the relatively benign adverse effect profile of the SSRIs in comparison to the TCAs allowed the investigators to titrate to the highest doses permitted in the ascending dose design studies that were typically used in the early studies with these drugs. This dose issue is one of the limitations of this approach in contrast to having data from the ideal study described at the beginning of this chapter.

TABLE 5.2 — COMPARISON OF THE PLACEBO-ADJUSTED INCIDENCE RATE (%) OF FREQUENT ADVERSE EFFECTS FOR SSRIS*

Item	Fluoxetine (n=1730, n=799)[1]	Fluvoxamine (n=222, n=192)[1]	Paroxetine (n=421, n=421)[1]	Sertraline (n=861, n=853)[1]
Headache	4.8	2.9	0.3	1.3
Nervousness[2]	10.3	7.6	4.9	4.4
Tremors	5.5	6.1	6.4	8.0
Insomnia	6.7	4.0	7.1	7.6
Drowsiness[3]	5.9	17.2	14.3	7.5
Fatigue[4]	5.6	6.2	10.3	2.5
Dizziness/lightheadedness	4.0	1.3	7.8	5.0
Vision disturbances	1.0	0	2.2	2.1
Nausea	11.0	25.6	16.4	14.3
Diarrhea	5.3	– 0.4	4.0	8.4
Dry mouth	3.5	1.8	6.0	7.0
Anorexia	7.2	8.6	4.5	1.2
Dyspepsia	2.1	3.2	0.9	3.2

Frequent micturation	1.6	0.6	2.4	0.8
Constipation	1.2	11.2	5.2	2.1
Sweating	4.6	-1.3	8.8	5.5
Respiratory[5]	5.8	-1.3	0.8	0.8
Palpitations[6]	-0.1	NA	1.5	1.9
Urinary retention[7]	—	NA	2.7	0.9

* Data for fluoxetine, paroxetine and sertraline is from reference 211; data for fluvoxamine is from reference 89. Incidence of each respective adverse effect for patients taking each drug minus the incidence for each drug's parallel placebo condition.

[1] The first value is the number of patients on that medication, while the second represents those treated in the parallel, placebo group.

[2] Nervousness is a composite of the following terms: nervousness, anxiety, agitation.

[3] Includes somnolence, sedation.

[4] Includes asthenia, myasthenia, hypokinesia.

[5] Includes respiratory disorder, upper respiratory infection, flu, dyspnea, pharyngitis, sinus congestion, oropharynx disorder.

[6] Includes tachycardia.

[7] Includes micturition disorder, difficulty with micturition, and urinary hesitancy.

NA = Not available

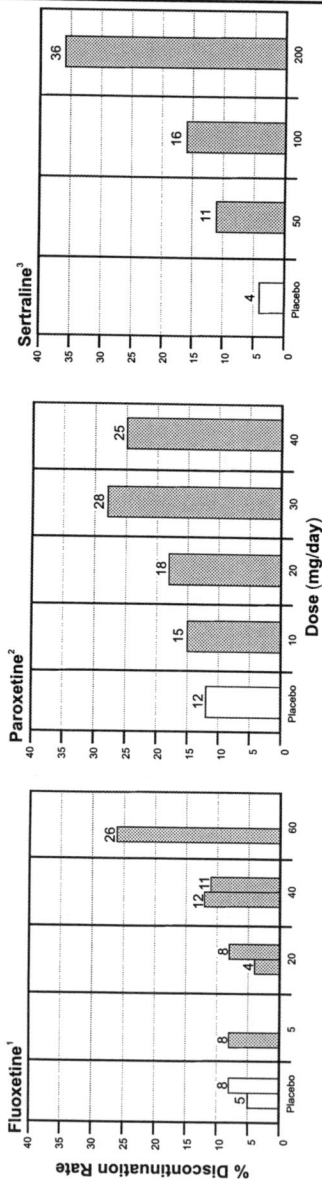

FIGURE 5.1 — DISCONTINUATION RATE DUE TO ADVERSE EVENTS AS A FUNCTION OF DOSE FOR THREE SSRIS*

* Comparable data from fixed dose studies has not been published for citalopram or fluvoxamine.

References: [1]283, [2]284; [280]; [3]85

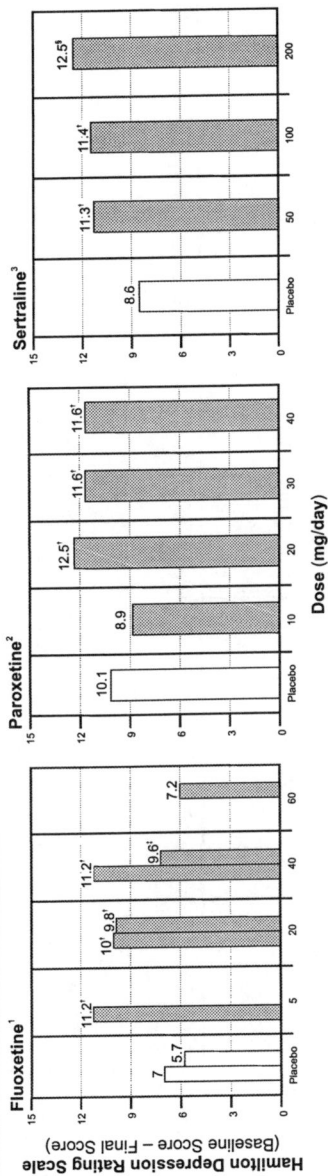

FIGURE 5.2 — ANTIDEPRESSANT EFFICACY AS A FUNCTION OF DOSE FOR THREE SSRIS*

* Comparable data from fixed dose studies has not been published for citalopram or fluvoxamine.

[†] $P < 0.05$
[‡] $P < 0.01$
[§] $P < 0.001$ compared to placebo

References: [1]283; [2]284; [3]280; [3]85

TABLE 5.3 — ADVERSE EVENTS FOR EACH SSRI THAT OCCURRED ≥ 1% MORE OFTEN THAN WITH OTHER SSRIS*			
Fluoxetine	**Fluvoxamine**	**Paroxetine**	**Sertraline**
• Nervousness/agitation/anxiety[†] • Respiratory complaints • Headache	• Nausea • Drowsiness • Constipation • Anorexia[†]	• Sexual dysfunction[†] • Frequent micturition • Asthenia/fatigue[†] • Dizziness • Sweating	• Loose stools • Tremors • Dry mouth

* Placebo-adjusted rates using the results of placebo-controlled, double-blind studies for each SSRI respectively. Based on analysis of data in Table 5.2.

† Dose-dependent adverse effects of SSRIs which can mimic symptoms of major depression.

NOTE: Insomnia is another dose-dependent, adverse effect of SSRIs and also can be a symptom of major depression. Insomnia is not shown above because its incidence as an adverse effect is virtually identical for fluoxetine, paroxetine and sertraline, but is lower for fluvoxamine (Table 5.2).

Nonetheless, the data in Table 5.2 is state-of-the-art and fortunately the dosing issue is somewhat mitigated by the fact that overdosage during the clinical trials was virtually universal with these drugs. With this caveat in mind, Table 5.3 lists specific adverse effects that have at least a 1% higher incidence rate on a specific SSRI in comparison to the other 3.

The SSRIs as a class also produce a variety of sexual dysfunction adverse effects, including anorgasmia and decreased libido (Table 5.4). Although an analysis of the clinical trial database for each SSRI suggests that fluvoxamine and fluoxetine are less likely to produce these effects than paroxetine and sertraline, clinical experience suggests that all SSRIs produce a comparable rate at their usually effective, minimum antidepressant dose.[130,280,296] One possible reason for the lower rates in the clinical trial databases for fluvoxamine and fluoxetine is that these two SSRIs were the first to be extensively studied and that unfamiliarity with this adverse effect may have contributed to an under-reporting of its occurrence. Again, the ideal study described at the beginning of this chapter would more convincingly answer this question; in the interim, clinicians will have to assess this matter using the available data and their clinical experience. Clearly, sexual dysfunction is an unintended effect that can apparently be produced by serotonin uptake inhibition.

Of importance, a number of the dose-dependent adverse effects produced by the SSRIs can mimic clinical depression (Tables 5.3 and 5.4). These include:

- Nervousness/agitation/anxiety
- Drowsiness or daytime tiredness
- Anorexia
- Fatigue
- Sexual dysfunction, such as decreased libido.

This fact has several implications. First, the emergence of such adverse effects at higher doses may in part

TABLE 5.4 — PLACEBO-ADJUSTED INCIDENCE (%) OF VARIOUS FORMS OF SEXUAL DYSFUNCTION ON FOUR SSRIS[1]

Adverse Effect	Fluoxetine (n=1730, n=799)[2]	Fluvoxamine (n=222, n=192)[2]	Paroxetine (n=421, n=421)[2]	Sertraline (n=1033, n=1033)[2]
Abnormal ejaculation/orgasm[3]		1.4	12.9	13.3
Other male gender disorders[4]			10.0	
Decreased libido	1.6		3.3	
Sexual dysfunction (male)	1.9			
Sexual dysfunction (female)				1.5
Female genital disorder[5]			1.8	
Menstrual disorder[6]				0.5
Painful menstruation	0.5			

1 Incidence is based on gender whenever appropriate. Placebo incidence on average for each of the above categories is under 0.5%.
2 The first value is the number of patients on that medication, while the second represents those treated in the parallel, placebo group.
3 Incidence based on number of male patients.
4 Includes anorgasmia, delayed orgasm, erectile dysfunction, impotence, and "sexual dysfunction."
5 Includes vaginitis.
6 Includes dysmenorrhea and menstrual complaints.

From references: 89, 211

account for the fact that the antidepressant response rate to the SSRIs tends to be lower on average at doses higher than the usually effective, minimum dose based on the result of fixed-dose studies (Figure 5.2). Second, physicians may misinterpret the emergence of such adverse effects as the need for higher doses and thus increase the dose unwittingly, worsening the situation. The late emergence of these effects as a result of gradual drug accumulation may be interpreted as the drug losing its effectiveness. This phenomenon is one reason the physician should ensure that the patient has had an adequate trial on the usually effective, minimum dose of each SSRI. For the same reason, the physician may also wish to consider a dose reduction rather than increase if the patient initially appeared to respond and then has a recurrence of symptoms. This phenomenon also is relevant to the potential role of therapeutic drug monitoring (TDM) with SSRIs which is discussed later in this section.

Efficacy — Acute

The major indication for the use of SSRIs is the treatment of major depression. There are 3 types of efficacy that are important in this condition:

- Acute amelioration of the depressive syndrome
- Maintenance of that improvement during the vulnerable period for a relapse
- Prophylactic treatment to prevent the occurrence of a new episode[92,150,151,233]

There is a variable amount of data for the various SSRIs on the first two uses and no systematic data for any of them on their ability to prevent recurrent episodes for a period greater than 1 year. The comparable data existing for these 2 uses in major depression does not reveal any difference among the SSRIs in terms of either the induction of acute response or maintenance of that response for a period up to 1 year (Table 5.5).

Before reviewing that data, it is important to note that the efficacy of SSRIs is not limited to major depression but extends to several other conditions including obsessive-compulsive disorder, panic disorder, and even conditions such as premature ejaculation.[156,199] The efficacy of these drugs in these other conditions appears to be due to their indirect serotonin agonism via serotonin uptake inhibition and hence is probably a class phenomenon. Different SSRIs have approval for several of these other indications in different countries, others have applications pending for such approval, and still others are in clinical testing in hopes of obtaining data that will support application for formal labeling for these conditions. Fluvoxamine is an example of vagaries of such approvals. It is formally labeled in the US for the treatment of obsessive-compulsive disorder but not for major depression even though it has that indication in many other countries. Since major depression is the principal, clinical use of these drugs and has the largest amount of comparative data, it will be the focus of this discussion of their comparative efficacy.

Two approaches were taken to compare the efficacy of the different SSRIs in terms of the acute relief of depressive symptoms. The first was a meta-analysis of the double-blind, placebo-controlled studies and the second was a comparison of the results of placebo controlled, fixed-dose studies. The latter is critical to determining whether there is a difference among the drugs in terms of their efficacy at the usually effective, minimum dose. Of necessity, these comparisons had to be limited to the SSRIs for which published data existed from such studies.

It was possible to do the meta-analysis with 4 of the 5 SSRIs: fluvoxamine, fluoxetine, paroxetine and sertraline.[226] The results of such studies with citalopram

91

TABLE 5.5 — SSRI VERSUS PLACEBO: RESPONSE RATE AND RELAPSE RATE

	Response Rate (%)[1]				Duration[†] (weeks)	Relapse Rate (%)[2-4]			
	SSRI	Placebo	Difference	P Value		Placebo	Drug	Difference	P Value
Fluoxetine	60	33	27	$< 10^{-13}$	52	57	26	31	< 0.01
Fluvoxamine	67	42	25	$< 10^{-2}$	NA	NA	NA	NA	NA
Paroxetine	65	36	29	$< 10^{-14}$	52	43	16	27	< 0.01
Sertraline	79	48	31	$< 10^{-11}$	44	46	13	33	< 0.001

The meta-analysis for response rate did not include citalopram. A relapse prevention study has been done with citalopram, but lasted 24 weeks rather than one year. Its results are discussed in the text. A relapse prevention study has not been published for fluvoxamine.

* Response defined as at least 50% decrease in depression symptom severity, as measured using a standard instrument.
† Duration of maintenance treatment follow-up.

From references: [1]226, [2]175, [3]375, [4]482

were not published in sufficient detail at the time of this meta-analysis to permit that SSRI to be included. Based on the results of this meta-analysis, each SSRI produces approximately a 60% overall response rate (ie, at least a 50% reduction in symptoms as a result of treatment) and a 30% higher response rate than a parallel, placebo control. This meta-analysis suggests that approximately the same percentage of patients with major depression respond to approximately the same degree to each of these 4 SSRIs. The data that has been published on citalopram suggests its efficacy is comparable.[174,177]

Double-blind, placebo-controlled, fixed-dose studies are the only way to determine the optimal dose of a drug and what is a comparably effective dose for different drugs in the same class (ie, having the same MOA mediating that outcome). Such studies have been done with all of the SSRIs, but the results have not been presented yet for the citalopram or fluvoxamine studies. Therefore, this analysis is of necessity limited to the studies with fluoxetine, paroxetine and sertraline (Figure 5.2).

Based on available studies, each of these 3 SSRIs have a flat-dose antidepressant-response curve meaning that they produce approximately the same average response rate at each dose above their usually effective, minimum dose over their clinically relevant dosing range (Figure 5.2). Based on these studies, the usually effective, minimum dose for fluoxetine and paroxetine is 20 mg/day and for sertraline 50 mg/day. Paroxetine was the only 1 of the 3 to include an ineffective dose, 10 mg/day.[80] In 1 study, fluoxetine (5 mg/day) was as effective as 20 mg/day on the Hamilton Depression Rating Scale but was not effective on other measures. This lack of robust effectiveness and the limited studies with fluoxetine 5 mg/day has been the basis for concluding that 20 mg/day is the optimal dose.[6] The conclusion that 50 mg/day of sertraline is its optimal dose based on its fixed-dose study is further supported by a review of its other efficacy studies.[229]

If anything, the response rate in the fixed-dose clinical trials tends to be lower at higher doses of fluoxetine and paroxetine. As mentioned above, one reason for this result may be the emergence of dose-dependent, adverse effects which mimic symptoms of major depression. Consistent with this explanation, the discontinuation rate due to adverse effects increases at higher doses for all 3 of these SSRIs (Figure 5.1).

Given the delayed onset of antidepressant response seen with SSRIs and other antidepressants, an increase in dropouts at higher doses will also bias against the response rate at higher doses since patients will be prone to discontinuing the trial before they may reasonably be expected to respond. Regardless of the reason, the decrease in the average magnitude of the antidepressant effect for fluoxetine and paroxetine reinforces the recommendation to ensure that the patient has had an optimal trial on the usually effective dose of the SSRIs before attempting a dose increase unless the physician uses a TDM approach to judge the adequacy of the dose in the patient as discussed later in this chapter.

The usually effective dose of fluvoxamine and citalopram have not been convincingly established due to the absence of published data from appropriately designed and executed fixed-dose studies. Nonetheless, a meta-analysis of the placebo-controlled studies with citalopram has been published in 2 separate publications.[174,177] The results of this meta-analysis suggest that citalopram also has a flat-dose antidepressant-response curve in terms of antidepressant efficacy.

Nevertheless, this meta-analysis is not an adequate substitute for publication of the fixed-dose studies. Its interpretation is compromised by the fact that the studies involve different criteria for subject selection, different designs, and different scales. Additionally, it is based on the data from only approximately 60% of the patients who were assigned to the citalopram treatment arms (ie, a selected group of patients who stayed on treatment for at least 4 weeks). A case was made using this meta-analysis that 20 mg/day of citalopram is the usually effective dose in patients who do not have severe and/or melancholic major depression. However, the published results of the 1 fixed-dose study with citalopram showed that 40 mg/day was statistically superior to placebo at weeks 3, 4 and 6 and superior to 20 mg/day at weeks 4 and 6 ($p < 0.05$), while 20 mg/day was not statistically superior to placebo at any time.[178] In contrast to the meta-analysis, the analysis of this fixed-dose study used the more conservative and more generally accepted "last observation carried forward" approach. Until the results of the other fixed-dose studies with citalopram are adequately presented, the results from the published, fixed-dose study serves as the basis for concluding that 40 mg/day is the usually effective, minimum dose for citalopram as shown in Table 3.7.

Returning to the fixed-dose studies with fluoxetine, paroxetine and sertraline, the magnitude of the antidepressant effect (ie, the absolute reduction in depressive symptoms as quantitated using the Hamilton Depression Rating Scale) was also virtually identical for these 3 SSRIs at their usually effective, minimum dose (Figure 5.2). These findings suggest that each of these drugs treats approximately the same percentage of patients to approximately the same extent at their respective minimally effective doses. Consistent with this finding is the fact that each of these SSRIs at these doses produces approximately a 70% to 80% inhibition of serotonin uptake using the platelet as a surrogate marker for the effect on the central serotonin neurons (Table 3.7). The plasma concentration of each SSRI at comparable antidepressant doses are consistent with the concentrations predicted to be needed to produce this magnitude of uptake inhibition based on the *in vitro* IC50 data.

Figure 5.3 further illustrates that the major effect on serotonin uptake inhibition with SSRIs occurs at the lower end of their clinically relevant dosing range using data from studies with sertraline as a representative SSRI.[223] In this study, normal volunteers were randomly assigned to 1 of 4 fixed-doses of sertraline. The plasma levels that they achieved and the degree of serotonin uptake inhibition that occurred on each of the 4 doses was measured. The platelet was used as a surrogate in lieu of measuring the effect of the drug on central serotonin neurons. As is apparent in Figure 5.3, 80% of serotonin uptake inhibition was achieved at plasma levels produced by the 50 mg/day dose. While both the plasma levels of the drug and the degree of serotonin uptake inhibition increased as expected with the higher fixed-doses, the higher levels at 200 mg/day were associated with only an additional 8% increase in serotonin uptake inhibition further reflecting the fact that majority of the effect had already occurred and the plateau portion of the dose-response curve had been reached. The fact that this dose-response curve is so similar to the dose-response curve for the antidepressant efficacy of the drug (ie, that is relatively flat above 50 mg/day) provides an heuristic explanation consistent with the presumed MOA for both effects being the result of the effect of sertraline on the serotonin uptake pump. The relationship illustrated in Figure 5.3 is not unique for sertraline but is simply illustrative of curves that can be drawn for any of the SSRIs which have been so studied. This phenomenon is again consistent with how these drugs were rationally developed.

All of the above observations raise serious questions about the widespread clinical practice of routinely using higher doses of SSRIs before there has been an

5

FIGURE 5.3 — RELATIONSHIP BETWEEN DAILY DOSE OF SERTRALINE, MEAN PLASMA LEVELS OF SERTRALINE, AND MEAN REDUCTION IN SEROTONIN UPTAKE BY PLATELETS AFTER 14 DAYS OF DRUG ADMINISTRATION AT ONE OF FOUR FIXED DOSES

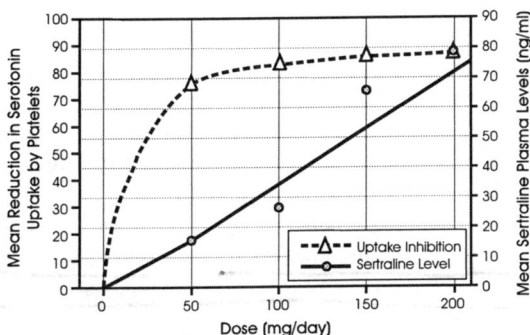

Reference: 223

adequate trial on their usually effective, minumum dose. The only double-blind, adequately powered study to test whether early nonresponders to an SSRI would benefit from a higher dose randomly assigned patients who had not responded after 3 weeks of treatment with fluoxetine 20 mg/day to either stay on 20 mg/day or be treated with 60 mg/day.[77] At the end of an additional 5 weeks of treatment, an equal number of patients had responded in both groups and the time course for response was also the same. This study is fully consistent with the flat-dose antidepressant-response curve and indicates that 3 weeks is not a sufficient trial to determine that the usually effective dose of this SSRI is inadequate for a patient. Parenthetically, fluoxetine is not the ideal SSRI for this type of study since the long half-lives of the parent drug and active metabolite may make a delayed response more likely than with the other more intermediate-lived SSRIs. Nonetheless, the data exists for this SSRI and not the others.

The reason to adequately test the antidepressant response to the usually effective, minumum dose is to optimize the tolerability of the drug and to avoid unintended effects on CYP enzymes (see Sections 7 and 8). While the effect on antidepressant response and serotonin uptake inhibition of the SSRIs has on average reached the plateau portion of their dose-response curve, that is not true for their discontinuation rate due to adverse effects (Figure 5.1) nor for the effects of specific SSRIs on specific CYP enzymes (eg, fluoxetine on CYP 2D6). Thus, the trade-off for using higher doses than necessary is to increase the degree of CYP enzyme inhibition produced, possibly the number of CYP enzymes inhibited and number and severity of dose-dependent adverse effects which can mimic major depression. All of these adverse consequences can occur with higher than the usually effective dose without improving antidepressant efficacy.

These observations also raise serious question about the widespread clinical practice of switching from one SSRI to another if the patient fails to respond to the first SSRI after a reasonable therapeutic trial. Conceivably, there is some as yet unidentified difference in the spectrum of antidepressant activity of these drugs, but the available data is not suggestive that a meaningful difference exists. There is certainly no compelling double-blind, placebo-controlled data to support this practice. It is clearly an important deficiency in our knowledge when faced with a patient who has not responded to a member of this class of drugs.

In addition to acute efficacy, fluoxetine, paroxetine and sertraline have been studied in terms of their ability to prevent a recurrence of a depressive episode in the 1-year interval following the induction of an acute response (Table 5.5). The design of these studies is similar so that the results can be reasonably compared: patients were brought into remission on the SSRI and after a period of several months of stabilization were randomly assigned in a double-blind fashion to either remain on the SSRI or be switched to placebo. As with acute efficacy, the results of these studies are amazingly consistent: continued treatment with each SSRI produced an approximately 30% reduction in the risk of relapse compared to the parallel, placebo control in the 1-year period of follow-up observation. A similar study was done with citalopram, but for 6 months rather than 1 year. Like the other 3 SSRIs, citalopram was superior to placebo having a 20.5% lower risk of relapse at that point.[179] That result is comparable to the result with the other 3 SSRIs at the same time point in the longer studies with those drugs. A relapse prevention study has not been published with fluvoxamine. The expectation is that it will be similarly effective.

Therapeutic Drug Monitoring

The discussion about the flat-dose antidepressant-response curve is not meant to imply that there are no patients who will benefit from a dose other than the usually effective, antidepressant dose. The phrase "on average" is key to that discussion. Like the effect on serotonin uptake inhibition (Figure 5.3) and specific CYP enzyme inhibition (Figure 8.3 and 8.4), the antidepressant effect and adverse effects of SSRIs must be concentration-dependent although the "signal-to-noise" problems in such research makes it difficult to show a strong correlation between these clinical effects and plasma drug levels.

Since the plasma levels achieved on the same dose of the same SSRI can differ among patients, there are undoubtably some patients who need a lower dose to achieve the concentration that usually occurs on the usually effective, antidepressant dose and, conversely, some patients need a higher dose to achieve the same levels. The problem is that it is obviously difficult to detect this fact using dose alone.

One approach to this problem is simply careful dose titration based on clinical assessment of response. However, there are several problems with this approach. First, there is no compelling data about what is an adequate duration to know that the usually effective dose is wrong for that specific patient. The only data on this issue indicates that 3 weeks is an inadequate trial for fluoxetine, but not what is an adequate trial for this or any other SSRI. Second, the clinician would have to be able to distinguish between dose-dependent, adverse effects that mimic depressive symptoms and the depressive symptoms themselves. The placebo response rate in clinical trials does not suggest that even experienced clinical investigators can consistently determine when a response is specifically treatment related. For these reasons, TDM can have a role in deciding whether a specific patient needs a dose other than the usually effective, minimum dose.

A few general comments may be helpful to put this discussion in perspective. Unlike TCAs, TDM with SSRIs will almost undoubtably never be a standard-of-care issue. The avoidance of serious toxicity is the overriding rationale for TDM. That is not an issue with the SSRIs in contrast to the TCAs. Due to their narrow therapeutic index, their potentially life-threatening toxicity, and wide interindividual variability in clearance, some patients on conventional antidepressant doses of TCAs can experience serious adverse consequences (eg, delirium, seizures, arrhythmias).[221] The avoidance of such toxicity primarily in patients who are deficient in CYP 2D6 function either due to genetics or concomitantly prescribed drugs (eg, fluoxetine, paroxetine) is the reason for obtaining a plasma level once early in the course of treatment with a TCA to permit a rational dose adjustment if needed.

A second and less pressing reason to use TDM is to increase efficacy and tolerability by adjusting the dose upward in patients who have rapid clearance to increase efficacy and downward in those with slow clearance to improve tolerability and thus efficacy.[221] This reason would be applicable to drugs like the SSRIs which have a sufficiently wide therapeutic index such that serious toxicity is not a concern, but nevertheless can produce a greater increase in adverse effects than an increase in efficacy on average at higher doses (Figures 5.1 and 5.2), especially since some of those adverse effects can be confused with lack or loss of efficacy (Table 5.3).

The problem is establishing the plasma levels of the various SSRIs that will produce the optimal balance of antidepressant efficacy and tolerability. One approach that has been used is to try to correlate plasma levels of the various SSRIs with antidepressant response in clinical trials. Such studies have been published with all of the SSRIs and have all failed to show a relationship between drug concentration and antidepressant response: citalopram,[31,79] fluoxetine,[232,142] fluvoxamine,[37,140] paroxetine,[158,269] and sertraline.[223] That is not surprising for many reasons including the "signal-to-noise" problem created by placebo response and the fact that these studies used doses at or above the usually effective, minimum dose. In other words, they examined the plateau portion of the dose-response curve where one would predict that there would be no relationship between concentration and response.

The concentration-dependent nature of antidepressant response with the SSRIs is apparent from the flat-dose antidepressant-response relationship and the fact that it parallels the dose- and concentration-dependent effect on serotonin uptake inhibition (Figure 5.3). This relationship is consistent with a minimum threshold concentration that produces approximately 70% serotonin uptake inhibition and exerts a step-function effect on antidepressant response. However, a study demonstrating such a relationship will have to focus on doses which produce concentrations both below this level and somewhat above, in contrast to the studies that have been done. Such a study will also have to involve hundreds of patients to overcome the "noise" in current antidepressant clinical trials research. The interested reader is referred to a previous paper that discusses the technical problems of doing such research in psychiatry.[230]

The ideal TDM study with the SSRIs described above will most likely never be done for cost and logistical reasons. There is no compelling incentive on the part of any government or private research sponsor to demonstrate the concentration-dependent nature of antidepressant response to SSRIs. In fact, the manufacturer may actually have a disincentive out of concern that the demonstration of such a relationship might be used to suggest that TDM is necessary with their medication and thus create a perception that may adversely impact the clinical acceptance of the drug.

In the absence of data from such an ideal TDM study, the fixed-dose studies can be used to estimate the optimal plasma level range as illustrated in Figure 5.4. Fixed-dose studies take advantage of group difference to establish the superiority of the drug over placebo. As illustrated in this figure, some patients will do as well on placebo as the best patient does on the drug at any dose, and some patients on the drug will do as poorly as any patient on placebo. In other words, there is complete overlap in the range of the response between the two groups. That is what is meant by the term, "noise," in these studies. The ability to

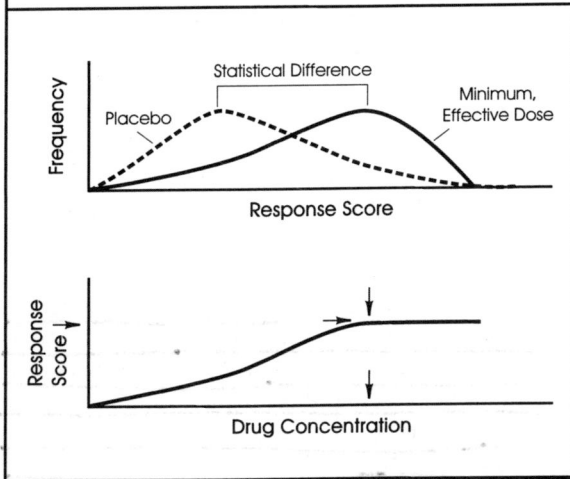

FIGURE 5.4 — ESTIMATED MINIMUM EFFECTIVE DRUG CONCENTRATION: AVERAGE PLASMA DRUG CONCENTRATION ACHIEVED IN THE GROUP TREATED WITH THE MINIMUM, EFFECTIVE DOSE

show a difference between drug and placebo is based on the fact that the curve for the drug-treated group is skewed to the responder side, whereas the curve of the placebo-treated group is skewed to the nonresponder side to a statistically significant extent The usually effective, minimum dose is the lowest dose that separates the drug from placebo. In the case of the SSRIs, it is also the best dose for most patients (Figure 5.2).

The usually effective dose defines an expected concentration range (Figure 5.4) based on the variability of the clearance of the drug in different patients. Since this dose on average separates drug treatment from placebo, the concentration that on average is achieved by this dose must also separate the drug from placebo. This concentration then is an estimate of the minimum desired concentration. Since higher doses on average increase adverse effects more than efficacy, the average plasma levels produced by those doses define the upper threshold where generally nuisance adverse effects outweigh additional therapeutic benefit. It would be ideal to have a low dose in the fixed-dose study that does not separate the drug from placebo because the concentration achieved by that dose will more convincingly establish the minimum threshold concentration. Such data exists for paroxetine (10 mg/day)[80] and possibly for citalopram (≤ 20 mg/day).[178] If that has not been established, then one does not know whether a lower threshold will actually be better on average in terms of the balance between efficacy and tolerability.

This information can help the clinician in the decision-making process. A patient may have failed on the usually effective, minimum dose because s/he is not responsive to this MOA or because plasma concentration of the drug is below the usually effective threshold due to an unusually rapid clearance of the drug in that patient. TDM can be used to provide information relevant to the latter possibility. If TDM reveals substantially lower plasma drug levels than would normally be expected for patients on this dose, the problem may be noncompliance or rapid clearance. In the former case, the physician could visit with the patient and determine what is leading to compromised compliance. In the event of rapid clearance, a trial of a higher dose will be more rational than switching to another SSRI or to another class of antidepressants. The goal will be to ensure that each patient receives a trial of a dose which will result in that patient achieving plasma drug levels that are usually therapeutic for that drug. If the patient has a level considerably above the range produced by the usually effective, minimum dose due to unusually slow clearance, then a dose reduction may be warranted to determine whether the less than optimal response is due to adverse effects that are mimicking depressive symptomatology.

The goal of this TDM approach is to aid rather than to dictate the dose adjustment. Such TDM data would have to be considered by the physician along with other factors specific to that patient such as clinical assessment of efficacy and tolerability. As stated above, TDM is clearly not a necessity with SSRIs. Their wide therapeutic index means that clinicians can titrate the dose over large ranges without concern about serious toxicity. Some physicians will, therefore, never use TDM with these drugs. Others may use this approach in nonresponders. A few might even wonder whether this TDM approach might have sufficient clinical and cost-effectiveness advantages to use it early in treatment as a routine aspect of treatment. The goal in this latter approach would be to reduce the time needed to determine whether the usually effective, minimum dose in that patient is producing the usually expected plasma levels in the patient. The potential advantages will be reducing the duration of the illness by being able to more rapidly make dose adjustments and by not erroneously concluding that the patient is not responsive to the drug when the problem is unusually rapid or slow clearance of the drug.

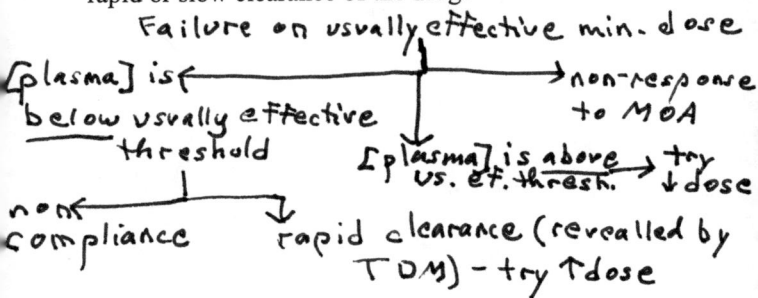

6   What Are the Clinically Relevant Pharmacokinetic Differences Among SSRIs?

While the serotonin selective reuptake inhibitors (SSRIs) were rationally developed to be similar in terms of avoiding effects on several neural sites of action (SOAs), they were not designed to be similar with regard to their pharmacokinetics. Not surprisingly, this area is one where there are clinically meaningful differences among these drugs.

Concentration-dependent Effects of SSRIs

The concentration-dependent effects of SSRIs are summarized in Table 6.1. Chapter 5 reviewed the data on the concentration-dependent nature of the effects of SSRIs in terms of the inhibition of the serotonin uptake pump, their antidepressant efficacy, and the incidence and severity of their serotonin-mediated adverse effects. The concentration-dependent inhibition of specific CYP enzymes by specific SSRIs will be presented in Sections 7 and 8. The concentration-dependent nature of these effects is the basis for the clinical importance of the pharmacokinetic differences among SSRIs (Table 6.2).

The only pharmacokinetic parameters shared by all the SSRIs is that they are relatively slowly, but completely, absorbed from the gut (ie, time to peak plasma concentration is 3 to 8 hours) and have large apparent volumes of distribution.[213] They differ with regard to:

TABLE 6.1 — CONCENTRATION-DEPENDENT EFFECTS OF SSRIS

- Serotonin uptake inhibition (eg, platelets)
- Antidepressant efficacy
- Incidence and severity of serotonin-mediated adverse effects
- Competitive inhibition of specific CYP enzymes

- Their protein binding
- Their metabolism including which CYP enzymes are principally responsible for their biotransformation
- Their half-lives
- Whether they have linear or nonlinear pharmacokinetics over their clinically relevant dosing range
- Whether they have active metabolites
- The effect of age and specific organ impairment on their elimination rates

Protein Binding

Fluoxetine, paroxetine and sertraline are highly protein bound (ie, > 95%).[213] In contrast, the protein binding of citalopram (50%) and fluvoxamine (77%) is considerably less.[94,199] High protein binding raises the possibility of displacement interaction with other highly protein bound drugs. However, SSRIs are weakly bound primarily to α1-acid glycoprotein. Perhaps for this reason, even the highly protein bound SSRIs have not been found to increase the free fraction of concomitantly administered drugs that are also highly protein bound.

TABLE 6.2 — PHARMACOKINETIC PARAMETERS RELEVANT TO THE USE OF SSRIS

Parameter	Citalopram	Fluoxetine	Fluvoxamine	Paroxetine	Sertraline
Autoinhibition[1]	No	Yes	Weakly yes	Yes	No
Half-life (in days)[2]	1.5	2 to 4[3] (7 to 15)[4]	0.5 to 1	1[3]	1
Time to steady-state (in days)	6 to 7	30 to 60[3,4]	3 to 5	4 to 5[4]	4 to 5
Dose-plasma level proportionality[5]	Yes	No[6]	Weakly no[6]	No	Yes
"Active" metabolite in terms of comparable *in vitro*[7] potency to parent drug for inhibiting specific CYP enzymes	Yes	Yes	Unknown	Yes	Yes

[1] See Table 6.4. [2] See Table 3.9. [3] At their usually effective, therapeutic dose (ie, 20 mg/day), but longer at higher doses due to autoinhibition. [4] Half-life ($t\frac{1}{2}$) of norfluoxetine which has virtually the same pharmacological profile as the parent drug and, hence, must be considered when calculating time to steady-state, time to maximal effect, and time to washout of effect. [5] See Table 6.5. [6] Based primarily on results summarized in Table 6.4; as seen in Table 6.5, there is scant published data measuring steady-state plasma levels at different doses for these two SSRIs. [7] See Table 8.7.

6

109

Metabolism

While some SSRIs can competitively inhibit specific CYP enzymes, the interaction between CYP enzymes and SSRIs is a two-way street. All of the SSRIs undergo extensive oxidative metabolism as a necessary step in their eventual elimination; however, different CYP enzymes mediate the metabolism of different SSRIs (Table 6.3). This knowledge is important because it forms the basis for understanding many of the other pharmacokinetic differences among the SSRIs. It is also important in terms of knowing whether concomitantly administered drugs can affect the clearance of specific SSRIs and hence their efficacy and tolerability. After all, SSRIs can be the target of pharmacokinetic drug-drug interactions as well as being the cause of such interactions.

Information about their metabolism varies substantially from one SSRI to another. The metabolism of citalopram and paroxetine have been the best characterized and sertraline is intermediate in terms of our knowledge; whereas there is considerably less information on the metabolism of fluoxetine and fluvoxamine, although for different reasons.

As reviewed in Section 2, citalopram is marketed as a racemic mixture and there are differences in the enantiomers in terms of their rate of metabolism. Racemic citalopram is metabolized by both CYP 2C19 and CYP 2D6 based on a study comparing the steady-state levels of citalopram, desmethylcitalopram, and didesmethylcitalopram in individuals who were extensive metabolizers of sparteine (ie, CYP 2D6) and mephenytoin (ie, CYP 2C19), and individuals who were poor metabolizers of either sparteine or mephenytoin respectively.[254] Both the total clearance of citalopram and the clearance of desmethylcitalopram were significantly slower in poor versus extensive

TABLE 6.3 — CYP ENZYME RESPONSIBLE FOR BIOTRANSFORMATION OF SSRIS

SSRI	CYP Enzyme Metabolized
Citalopram	2C19 mediates initial step, then 2D6
Fluoxetine*	2D6, partially responsible; remainder not established
Fluvoxamine	Not known
Paroxetine*	2D6, principal P450
Sertraline	3A3/4 responsible for demethylation

* The inhibition of this enzyme is responsible for nonlinear pharmacokinetics of paroxetine and at least partially for the nonlinear pharmacokinetics of fluoxetine.

6

metabolizers of mephenytoin (ie, deficient in CYP 2C19) while the demethylation clearance of desmethylcitalopram was significantly lower in poor versus extensive metabolizers of sparteine (ie, deficient in CYP 2D6). Both of these CYP enzymes exhibit considerable genetic polymorphism in specific populations: approximately 5% to 10% of white populations in western Europe and North America are genetically deficient in CYP 2D6[84,265] whereas 20% of Orientals are genetically deficient in CYP 2C19.[104,152] The fact that citalopram is dependent on these 2 enzymes will be expected to increase the interindividual variability in plasma levels of this drug.

Although fluvoxamine was one of the first SSRIs developed, it was developed before the technology existed to readily identify which CYP enzyme(s) was responsible for its biotransformation. Hence, there have been no formal studies examining which CYP enzymes are responsible for its biotransformation. This is unfortunate since the biotransformation of fluvoxamine is extensive and occurs mostly by oxidation.[198] Only negligible amounts of fluvoxamine are excreted unchanged in the urine. Eleven different metabolites have been identified in urine. However, a plot of the areas under curve (AUCs) of fluvoxamine in nearly 100 individuals did not reveal bimodality in distribution as would be expected if CYP 2D6 or CYP 2C19 were the rate-limiting enzyme.[73] However, smokers have a 23% reduction in fluvoxamine compared to nonsmokers, suggesting a possible role for CYP 1A2 in fluvoxamine metabolism.[275] The fact that fluvoxamine plasma levels are somewhat higher after multiple doses than after a single dose is also partially consistent with the fact that fluvoxamine can be metabolized by CYP 1A2 since fluvoxamine inhibits this enzyme. However, the nonlinearity in its plasma levels are not as great as would be predicted based on its effects on other CYP 1A2 substrates such as theophylline.

Knowledge about fluoxetine metabolism is also limited in part because such investigations are complicated by several factors:

- First, fluoxetine is marketed as a racemic mixture like citalopram.
- Second, it is *N*-demethylated to norfluoxetine, which is also chiral as discussed in Section 2.
- Third, fluoxetine and particularly norfluoxetine are slowly cleared (ie, extended half-lives).
- Fourth, both inhibit multiple CYP enzymes to varying degrees at clinically relevant concentrations and are known to inhibit their own metabolism presumably by inhibiting the responsible CYP enzymes. This matter is further complicated by the fact that the relative potency for such inhibition can vary between the enantiomers of both fluoxetine and norfluoxetine.

Thus, the knowledge about which CYP enzyme mediates the metabolism of fluoxetine is limited but will be summarized below to the extent possible.

The N-demethylation of both enantiomers of fluoxetine is probably at least in part metabolized by the same CYP enzyme(s) based on the results of an *in vitro* study showing a reasonable correlation between the rates at which human liver microsomes catalyze this reaction.[267] The R-fluoxetine was metabolized about 50% faster, which is consistent with reports of higher levels of S-fluoxetine in individuals on the drug.[18,267]

There are probably multiple CYP enzymes involved in the metabolism of fluoxetine at different concentrations, accounting for the nonlinear pharmacokinetics of the drug. As higher affinity enzymes become inhibited, lower affinity enzymes become relevant as the concentration of the drug increases. There is evidence suggesting a role for both CYP 2D6 and CYP 3A3/4. First, the metabolism of fluoxetine cosegregates with the CYP 2D6 polymorphism.[7,24] N-demethylation of fluoxetine positively correlates with CYP 2D6 levels in human microsomes, but is inhibited only 20% by quinidine and 27% by antisera to CYP 2D6 and does occur in human microsomes lacking the CYP 2D6 enzyme.[18,267] The fact that the N-demethylation of fluoxetine is autoinhibited at higher concentration suggests that this step is mediated at least in part by another CYP enzyme which is more weakly inhibited than CYP 2D6, such as CYP 3A3/4, 2C19, 2C9/10 or another CYP enzyme.

Paroxetine is metabolized principally to an intermediate, which is then conjugated and eliminated.[141] Two CYP enzymes mediate this reaction. There is ample evidence that at low paroxetine concentrations, this enzyme is CYP 2D6. First, enzyme activity at low concentrations of paroxetine cosegregates with the sparteine polymorphism and *in vitro* is responsible for approximately 75% of the activity in CYP 2D6 extensive metabolizers.[252,253] Second, this activity is inhibited by quinidine and by paroxetine itself, which are both known inhibitors of CYP 2D6.[32,252] The second CYP enzyme has a much lower affinity for paroxetine. It is responsible for 25% of the *in vitro* metabolism of paroxetine in CYP 2D6 extensive metabolizers at low concentrations but is the primary enzyme in CYP 2D6 poor metabolizers and in extensive metabolizers at higher concentrations.[253] This low affinity enzyme has not been identified but may be inhibited by cimetidine,[16,111] may decline in efficiency with age,[253] and may be induced by some anticonvulsants.[8]

While paroxetine is principally metabolized by CYP 2D6 at low concentrations, it also inhibits this enzyme in a concentration-dependent manner (see Section 8). Hence, this pathway becomes saturated at higher concentrations and paroxetine elimination becomes dependent on the lower affinity, but higher capacity, enzyme. The relative roles of these two enzymes in the metabolism of paroxetine is the apparent explanation for why paroxetine has nonlinear pharmacokinetics including a half-life of 10 hours after a single 20 mg dose, but a half-life of almost 24 hours after multiple doses of 20 mg/day.[141]

Sertraline, like the other SSRIs, is mainly eliminated by oxidative metabolism and the dominant metabolite is *N*-desmethylsertraline.[288] Several observations rule out a major role for CYP 2D6 in the metabolism of sertraline. First, there is no evidence of a bimodal distribution of plasma drug levels in populations of northern European extraction. Second, sertraline has linear pharmacokinetics even up to doses of 200 mg/day in terms of:

- No change in half-life from single dose to multiple dose
- No change in half-life over its full dosing range
- Proportional changes in plasma levels of both sertraline and desmethylsertraline with dose increases

PAXIL

- No change in the ratio of sertraline to desmethyl-sertraline[288]

These findings are not consistent with the conversion of sertraline to desmethylsertraline and its eventual elimination's being substantially dependent on CYP 2D6 since sertraline at a dosage of 150 mg/day does produce approximately a 50% to 65% increase in the plasma levels of the CYP 2D6 substrate, desipramine.[153,298] Also, an immediate switch from fluoxetine to sertraline exerts only a modest effect on sertraline and desmethylsertraline levels under conditions that produce a 400% increase in the levels of the desipramine. Third, the *in vitro* conversion of sertraline to desmethylsertraline correlates more with CYP 3A3/4 activity ($r = 0.93$) than with CYP 2D6 activity.[209] Therefore, higher and lower doses, respectively, of sertraline may be necessary when it is used in combination with drugs that induce (eg, carbamazepine and phenytoin) and inhibit (eg, ketoconazole) CYP 3A3/4.

The CYP enzymes responsible for the subsequent biotransformation of desmethylsertraline have not been well characterized. Several observations suggest that there is more than one potential pathway for the further biotransformation of sertraline prior to its elimination and that these pathways may be mediated by more than 1 CYP enzyme. Several different metabolites have been characterized in the plasma and/or urine of individuals receiving sertraline. Additionally, sertraline is excreted approximately equally in the feces and urine, suggesting that there is more than one metabolite.

Metabolites

There has been considerable discussion about whether the different SSRIs have "active" metabolites. One problem is that these discussions often do not begin with a definition of what is meant by the term "active" and how such activity was assessed. The two primary metabolites of fluvoxamine reportedly are not capable of inhibiting the serotonin uptake pump,[274] but no studies have been done on the effect of its numerous metabolites on specific CYP activity.

Fluoxetine has a metabolite that is as potent and more selective than the parent drug in terms of the inhibition of the serotonin uptake pump (Table 3.8). Since this metabolite has an unusually extended half-life (ie, 7 to 15 days), its level and hence indirect serotonin agonistic effects take time to fully develop and then persist for an extended interval after the fluoxetine is discontinued. Norfluoxetine is also more active than fluoxetine as an inhibitor of CYP 3A3/4 and equal to fluoxetine as an inhibitor of CYP 2D6 (Table 8.7). Plasma levels of norfluoxetine correlate with the magnitude and duration of the inhibition of both of these enzymes following fluoxetine administration.[112,219]

As with fluvoxamine, there are apparently no paroxetine metabolites capable of inhibiting the serotonin uptake pump, but the M2 metabolite is a potent inhibitor of CYP 2D6 (Table 8.7). There is no data on what plasma levels of this metabolite could be expected in the normal population or any of the special populations discussed later in this section.

Desmethylsertraline is 1/10th to 1/25th as potent as sertraline at inhibiting the serotonin uptake pump (Table 3.8). Since its concentrations are only 1.5 times higher than the parent drug under clinically relevant dosing conditions,[219] it would be predicted to contribute only 6% to 15% (ie, 1.5 times higher levels times 1/10th to 1/25th the potency) to the serotonin uptake inhibitory effects that would occur in patients on sertraline under clinically relevant dosing conditions. The magnitude of this contribution is probably too small to be clinically meaningful in most situations. However, desmethylsertaline like the major metabo-

116

lites of fluoxetine and paroxetine is virtually equipotent to the parent SSRI as an inhibitor of specific CYP enzymes (Table 8.7). Hence, it would be expected to contribute to the magnitude of such an effect. Since its half-life (62 to 104 hours) is longer than that of the parent drug, it would also be expected to prolong the duration of the effect, but not to the extent that norfluoxetine does.[288] The clinical impact of this fact is mitigated by the relatively weak inhibitory effect of sertraline and desmethylsertraline on specific CYP enzymes.

Linear Versus Nonlinear Pharmacokinetics

Citalopram and sertraline show linear pharmacokinetics (ie, changes in drug concentration proportional to the change in dose). In contrast, fluvoxamine, fluoxetine and paroxetine have nonlinear pharmacokinetics (Tables 6.4 and 6.5). The evidence for nonlinearity with fluvoxamine and fluoxetine primarily comes from the observation that their half-lives are substantially longer after multiple dose administration than after single dose administration (Table 6.4). The same observation also holds for paroxetine, but in addition, there is good evidence that under steady-state conditions, the half-life of paroxetine is progressively longer at higher doses.[141]

The nonlinearity of paroxetine is also apparent based on the fact that paroxetine plasma levels increase disproportionately with the dose increases (Table 6.5). In contrast, there is a linear relationship between dose and plasma drug level increases with both citalopram and sertraline (Table 6.5). Although fluoxetine has been the most extensively-used SSRI and fluvoxamine has been the longest-used SSRI, there are minimal data on what plasma drug levels can be reasonably expected at different doses administered long enough to achieve

TABLE 6.4 — CHANGE IN HALF-LIFE ($t_{\frac{1}{2}}$) AS A FUNCTION OF MULTIPLE DOSE ADMINISTRATION

SSRI	Single-dose $t_{\frac{1}{2}}$	Multiple-dose $t_{\frac{1}{2}}$	% Change
Citalopram[1]	33 hours	33 hours	—
Fluoxetine[2]	1.9 days	5.7 days*	↑ 300
Fluvoxamine[3]	15 hours	22 hours	≈ ↑ 50
Paroxetine[4]	10 hours†	21 hours	↑ 200
Sertraline[5]	26 hours	26 hours	—

* Only the effect on $t_{\frac{1}{2}}$ of fluoxetine is published.

† Paroxetine has the shortest half-life of any SSRI in terms of single dose which may increase the risk of withdrawal reactions on this drug. Tapering the drug rather than abrupt discontinuation should minimize such a reaction.

References: [1]146, [2]23, [3]234, [4]141, [5]288

steady-state. Undoubtedly, the long half-life of fluoxetine has discouraged such studies. It would require almost 1 year to determine the steady-state plasma levels of fluoxetine and norfluoxetine that could be achieved in the same individual on the 4 different doses that comprise its clinically relevant dosing range (ie, 20 to 80 mg/day).

Nonlinearity has the potential to be clinically significant with these SSRIs for several reasons. While fixed-dose studies with these drugs suggest that generally higher doses do not produce a greater antidepressant effect, physicians frequently try higher doses when the response has been suboptimal. Due to nonlinearity, the concentration-dependent effects of fluvoxamine, fluoxetine and paroxetine will be expected to increase disproportionally with higher doses;

that will not be expected with citalopram or sertraline. This knowledge can be helpful to the clinician in terms of what to expect with higher than usual doses of these different SSRIs. The dose-dependent (ie, concentration-dependent) effects of the SSRIs are reviewed in Section 5.

Half-life

Considerable variability among the SSRIs exists with regard to half-life (Table 6.2). The half-life of fluvoxamine is 15 to 22 hours.[73] For this reason, and to reduce the incidence and severity of nausea, it is generally administered in equally divided doses twice a day. The half-lives of citalopram, paroxetine and sertraline allow them to be administered once a day (Table 6.2). Fluoxetine and its active metabolite, norfluoxetine, have unusually extended half-lives for orally administered drugs: 2 to 4 days for fluoxetine and 7 to 15 days for norfluoxetine (Table 6.2). Because of the extended half-lives, this drug can be administered as infrequently as once a week and still reach stable steady-state levels.

Figure 6.1 provides a graphic illustration of the difference in duration of drug administration needed to reach steady-state and the time to 95% washout following drug discontinuation for fluoxetine and norfluoxetine versus the other SSRIs. Due to this extended period, the magnitude of any concentration-dependent effect of fluoxetine will take several weeks to be achieved and will persist for several weeks after it has been discontinued. The clinical consequences may be either desirable or undesirable depending on the specific situation. Such an extended half-life might provide an added measure of safety against possible relapse if the patient were intermittently noncompliant. While this proposal has theoretical appeal, it was not substantiated by the relapse prevention studies re-

TABLE 6.5 — EFFECTS OF DOSE AND AGE ON THE PLASMA LEVELS OF SSRIs

SSRI	Age (yrs)	Dose (mg/day) Plasma Level (ng/ml)				Dose Effect*	Age Effect†
Citalopram		5	20	25	50		
	< 65[1]	12	47‡	58	120	NC	
	> 65[2]	NA	109	NA	NA		↑ 133%
Fluoxetine		*20	40	60			
	< 65[3]	200	NA	NA		?	
	> 65[3]	NA	NA	NA			?
Fluvoxamine		50	100	200			
	< 65[4]	NA	93	250		↑ 25%?	
	> 65[5]	NA	62	NA			↓ 33%

		20	30	40	
Paroxetine					
	< 65[6]	49	86	129	↑ 25%
	> 65[6]	79	147	228	↑ 50% to 90%
Sertraline					
	< 65[7,8]	15§	29§	68§	NC
	> 65[8]	NA	NA	90	↑ 37%§

NA = Not available; NC = No change

* (Plasma level on dose [x + n] divided by plasma level on dose X) divided by (dose [X + n] divided by dose X) minus 1, or Δ change in plasma level ÷ Δ change in dose minus 1 expressed as %.

† (Plasma level for the elderly group divided by plasma level for the younger age group) minus 1 expressed as %.

‡ This result was extrapolated from the other values based on the linearity of citalopram plasma levels in this age group over this dose range.

§ These results are for males only. These results overestimate the effect of age since young males develop lower plasma levels on sertraline than do young females or older males or females. The values for young females at 20 mg/day is 104 ng/ml, which is essentially the same as for older males and females.

References: [1]31, [2]95, [3]Table 3.7, [4]73, [5]90, [6]141, [7]223, [8]243

viewed in Section 5 (Table 5.3). Instead, these studies show remarkably similar results for fluoxetine, paroxetine and sertraline versus a parallel placebo control. For the same theoretical reason, a slower onset of antidepressant efficacy may be expected with fluoxetine versus the other SSRIs, but there is no convincing data to support that proposal. While data are lacking on the above points, there are compelling data that the full magnitude of fluoxetine-induced inhibition of CYP 2D6 and 3A3/4 is not achieved until steady-state has been reached, and that full recovery of enzyme activity is not achieved until fluoxetine and norfluoxetine have fully washed out of the body.[112,219] These points are clinically important because the gradual accumulation and washout can affect the concentration of a concomitantly prescribed drug administered to a patient taking fluoxetine or recently discontinued from fluoxetine therapy. The extended half-life also is responsible for the long interval of washout that is recommended before initiating treatment with a monoamine oxidase inhibitor (MAOI) following fluoxetine discontinuation. At present, there is no good explanation for the unusually long half-life of norfluoxetine.

The half-life of paroxetine is a function of its plasma drug level. Following a single 20 mg dose, paroxetine has a half-life of 10 hours (Table 6.4). Paroxetine does not reach a half-life of 20 hours until steady-state has been reached on 20 mg/day (Table 6.4) because paroxetine inhibits CYP 2D6, which is the CYP enzyme responsible for its biotransformation. When paroxetine levels fall after this drug is discontinued, its clearance rate increases as the inhibition of the enzyme is decreased. Thus, paroxetine and fluvoxamine are more quickly cleared from the body than the other SSRIs.

Rapid clearance may explain the increased incidence of withdrawal reactions seen after these 2 SSRIs

122

PAXIL
LUVOX

FIGURE 6.1 — TIME TO STEADY-STATE AND TIME TO 95% WASHOUT

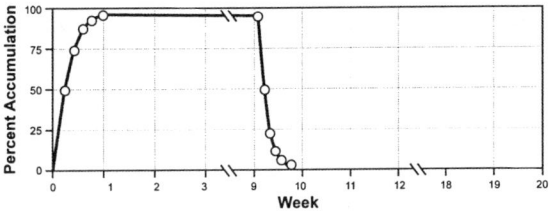

Citalopram (slightly longer)
Fluvoxamine (slightly shorter)
Paroxetine (at 20 mg/day)
Sertraline (across dosing range)

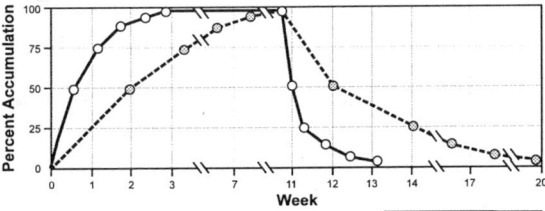

Fluoxetine
Norfluoxetine (at 20 mg/day)

Reference: 217

are discontinued in comparison to the other SSRIs. Certainly, such withdrawal syndrome would be highly unlikely with fluoxetine due to its extended half-life. If such a reaction were to occur after abrupt SSRI discontinuation, reinstituting the drug and more gradual tapering will commonly handle the problem. This approach may be taken prophylactically with fluvoxamine and paroxetine, particularly if the patient previously had problems with abrupt discontinuation or if the patient has been on higher than the usually effective, minimum dose.

Effect of Age and Gender on Clearance

Although the reasons have not been elucidated, there is considerable difference among the SSRIs with regard to changes in apparent clearance of specific SSRIs in the physically healthy "young old" (ie, in these studies, most of the "old" individuals were between 65 and 75 years of age) versus younger healthy individuals (Table 6.5). Plasma levels of citalopram and paroxetine are approximately 100% higher in the elderly compared with the young.[95,141] Fluvoxamine has no apparent change in its metabolism as a function of age;[73,234,285] however, recent data suggest males develop plasma levels 40% to 50% lower than females with the magnitude of the effect possibly being greater at lower doses.[118] The basis for this gender effect has not been established. Fluoxetine has not been adequately studied, but data from clinical trials suggest that plasma levels of fluoxetine plus norfluoxetine can be twice as high in the elderly compared to the young.[86,159] There is an age by gender interaction for sertraline with its plasma levels being 35% to 40% higher in elderly females versus young males; however, sertraline plasma levels do not differ between elderly females and elderly males or young females.[288]

There are at least two reasons why these age related changes in plasma drug levels can be clinically important:

- First, it will be predicted to increase treatment limiting adverse effects in the elderly since the discontinuation rate for SSRIs due to adverse effects is dose-dependent and, hence, concentration dependent.
- Second, the inhibition of specific CYP enzymes by specific SSRIs is concentration dependent;

hence, the elderly will be expected to experience a greater degree of inhibition on average than younger patients given the same dose of the same SSRI. The apparent order of the age effect from most to least appears to be citalopram > paroxetine ≥ fluoxetine (probably, although not well studied) > sertraline ≥ fluvoxamine (Table 6.5).

The latter issue is important since the elderly are more likely to be on concomitant therapy and more sensitive to any adverse consequences produced by elevation of the levels of such coadministered drugs. This phenomenon is particularly relevant to fluoxetine and fluvoxamine due to the number of CYP enzymes inhibited by these 2 SSRIs, which will be reviewed in Sections 7 and 8.

Effect of Specific Organ Impairment on Clearance

As discussed above, all of the SSRIs are dependent on oxidative metabolism for their elimination, and the resultant polar metabolites are primarily excreted via the urine. Based on these facts, significant impairment in liver, renal and cardiac function will be expected to affect the levels of either the parent drug and/or its metabolites for each of the SSRIs.

Appreciable impairment in liver function and/or size can slow the individual's ability to biotransform drugs and thus result in greater drug accumulation per dose prescribed. Reduced renal function generally leads to the increased accumulation of polar metabolites that may be pharmacologically active, either in a way similar to or different from the parent drug. The accumulation of those metabolites can appreciably alter the patient's response to the medication, including the risk of adverse effects. Significant reduction in

125

left ventricular function will cause a reduction in hepatic and renal arterial blood flow, which is another important determinant of both hepatic- and renal-mediated clearance of drugs. For these reasons, impairment in the function of these organs can significantly alter a patient's response to what is a usually therapeutic dose of a medication. The effect of specific organ impairment on the clearance of specific SSRIs has been studied to varying degrees with the different SSRIs.

Based on single-dose studies, the half-lives of all the SSRIs are approximately doubled in individuals with cirrhosis compared to physically healthy individuals (Table 6.6). Since the clearance of fluoxetine and paroxetine, to a substantial degree, and fluvoxamine, to a more modest degree, is prolonged when going from a single dose to multiple doses (Table 6.4), these single-dose studies in patients with cirrhosis are likely an underestimate of the magnitude of the effect of such impairment on the clearance of these SSRIs. As with the elderly, the elevated levels of specific SSRIs will translate into greater inhibition of specific CYP enzymes in this medically ill population.

The data on the effect of renal disease (Table 6.7) are even more limited than with cirrhosis particularly because the effect should principally be an increase in plasma levels of more polar metabolites, but the studies that have been done have focused only on the parent drug. In a single-dose study of paroxetine (30 mg) in individuals with renal impairment, the plasma AUC and Cmax were significantly increased.[281] Since the polar paroxetine metabolite, M2, is a potent inhibitor of CYP 2D6, accumulation of this metabolite may be relevant to the increase in paroxetine plasma levels in renally impaired individuals and also in the elderly since renal function decreases with age. The single-dose pharmacokinetics of fluvoxamine,[234] fluoxe-

TABLE 6.6 — EFFECT OF LIVER DISEASE ON SSRI METABOLISM AND PHARMACOKINETICS

Product	Average Half-life	
	Healthy Volunteers*	Cirrhosis Patients
Citalopram[1]	1.5 days	3.5 days
Fluoxetine[2]	2 days	7 days
Fluvoxamine[3]	15 hours	24 hours
Norfluoxetine[2]	7 days	12 days
Paroxetine[4]	12 hours	20 hours
Sertraline[5]	1 day	2 days

* It must be remembered that interindividual variability is high and that half-lives of fluoxetine, fluvoxamine and paroxetine are usually higher after multiple doses than after a single dose.

References: [1] 13, [2] 246, [3] 234, [4] 68, [5] 288

6

TABLE 6.7 — EFFECT OF RENAL IMPAIRMENT ON PHARMACOKINETICS OF SSRIs (SINGLE DOSE)

SSRI	Renal Impairment
Citalopram	Not available
Fluvoxamine	No effect[1]
Fluoxetine	No effect[2]
Sertraline	No effect[3]
Paroxetine	100-150% in plasma levels with GFR < 30 ml/min[4]

References: [1] 234, [2] 11, [3] 281, [4] 78

tine,[111] and sertraline[281,288] are similar in individuals with renal failure versus in healthy volunteers. As discussed above, single-dose studies with fluoxetine, and to a lesser extent with fluvoxamine, should be cautiously interpreted since the nonlinear pharmacokinetics of these drugs observed in healthy individuals (Tables 6.4 and 6.5) may well be increased in individuals with such organ impairment.

There have been no studies of the effect of significant left ventricular pump impairment on the clearance of any SSRI. In the absence of data, it would be prudent to use conservative dosing in such patients for the same reasons as discussed with hepatic and renal impairment.

The disease-related changes in the clearance rates of the SSRIs have several clinically important implications. Patients with such organ impairment will need lower doses to achieve the same plasma drug levels that occur in healthy individuals on the usually effective, minimum dose. Hence, a dose reduction will be appropriate for such individuals to compensate for the reduction in their clearance; otherwise, they will be at increased risk for having more of the dose-dependent adverse effects of the SSRIs and a poorer antidepressant responses. Additionally, these patients will be at increased risk for pharmacokinetic drug-drug interactions. Since inhibition of specific CYP enzymes produced by specific SSRIs is concentration-dependent (see Section 8), the higher levels that will occur in these patients without an appropriate dose adjustment will result in a greater degree of enzyme inhibition. The hepatic and cardiac impairment may also make these patients more sensitive to the enzymes inhibiting effects of these drugs (ie, a greater degree of enzyme inhibition may occur in these individuals than those with normal organs at the same concentration of the SSRI). There are no data on this matter because the formal pharmacokinetic drug interaction studies with the SSRIs have been done in healthy individuals with normal organ function.

These issues are important because these patients, due to their comorbid medical illnesses, are likely to be on multiple medications and at greater risk for a drug-drug interaction. Moreover, their medical illnesses may make them more susceptible to any adverse effects arising out of such an interaction. Being aware of these considerations can help the physician make a prudent choice with regard to SSRI selection and dose adjustment for a specific patient based on whether and to what degree one or more organ(s) is impaired, what other medications the patient is taking, and the overall health status of the patient.

6

7   Why Are CYP Enzymes Important When Considering SSRIs?

Cytochrome P450 (CYP) enzymes may be termed an "overnight discovery" a billion years in the making (Table 7.1). Only recently have we begun to understand the important role these enzymes play in determining a patient's response to pharmacotherapy. The inhibition of specific CYP enzymes is also the major distinguishing characteristic among SSRIs. Such inhibition produces the potential for specific pharmacokinetic drug interactions between specific SSRIs and concomitantly administered drugs dependent on specific CYP enzymes for their elimination. This section will provide the background information of how our understanding of these enzymes has evolved and their significance relative to the optimal care of patients.

Our knowledge of oxidative metabolism in the body and the role played by CYP enzymes has been relatively short, but has rapidly expanded, particularly

---

TABLE 7.1 — UNINTENDED TARGETS OF SOME SSRIS: CYP ENZYMES

- Evolved over 1 billion years ago
- Expressed in multiple tissues
- Highest concentration in hepatocytes
- Located in:
  - Mitochondria: steroidogenic CYP enzymes
  - Endoplasmic reticulum: xenobiotic CYP enzymes
- Mediate primarily oxidative metabolism

References: 105, 115, 116, 183-185, 187

---

over the last 10 years (Table 7.2). It was only about 100 years ago that drug metabolism was generally accepted to occur in the body. The pigments we now recognize to be multiple, different enzymes were identified approximately 50 years ago and named cytochrome P450 (CYP) due to their ability to absorb light at a frequency of 450 nm. The first gene to code for a specific CYP enzyme was isolated approximately 10 years ago. Due to the advances made possible by molecular biology, we can now study the effects of specific CYP enzymes on specific drugs and vice versa. We are currently "backfilling" our knowledge concerning which CYP enzymes are responsible for the metabolism of drugs.

Although our knowledge is relatively recent, the ancestral CYP enzyme from which all of the current ones evolved came into existence over 1 billion years ago, which underscores the biological importance of these enzymes to organisms, including man.[106,107] They are heme-containing monoxygensase enzymes responsible for much of the oxidative metabolism occurring in the body.[105]

Once the genes that code for specific CYP enzymes were isolated, they could be used to produce the enzymes in purified form — their amino acid sequence could then be determined. This has now been accomplished for all of the human CYP enzymes.

Using this information, a classification system has been developed based on the degree of structural similarities between different enzymes (ie, amino acid sequence homology).[187] The rationale for such a classification system is that the more similar the structure, the closer the enzymes are both phylogenetically and functionally (ie, function follows structure). The CYP enzymes are grouped into families designated by the first number. All enzymes in a family have at least 40% amino acid sequence homology. They are further grouped into subfamilies designated by an alpha-

TABLE 7.2 — HISTORY OF OUR KNOWLEDGE OF BIOTRANSFORMING ENZYMES

Knowledge	Time
Concept of entgiftung (detoxification) was appreciated	End of the 19th century
Correlation of some drug effects with *in vitro* metabolizing enzyme activities	1920s-40s
Induction of such enzymes possible	1940s-50s
Membrane bound cytochrome-CO complex discovered, named "cytochrome P450," and biochemically characterized	1950s-60s
Three hundred substances identified to induce their metabolism or that of foreign and endogenous substances	Mid-1960s
Role of mRNA and protein synthesis identified in induction process and purification of multiple P450 proteins accomplished, making polyclonal and monoclonal antibody studies possible	1970s
Identification of specific P450 genes using DNA cloning techniques	Mid-1980s to present

Reference: 218

bet letter. All enzymes in the same subfamily have at least 55% amino acid sequence homology. The last number designates the gene that codes for a specific enzyme. Table 7.3 shows all of the human CYP enzymes grouped into families and subfamilies.

These enzymes are divided into two major groups (Table 7.4):
- "Steroidogenic" CYP enzymes
- "Xenobiotic" CYP enzymes

The former are phylogenetically older, occurring in even single cell organisms. They are located in the mitochondria of cells and are responsible for the syn-

TABLE 7.3 — HUMAN CYP ENZYMES AS CLASSIFIED BY FAMILY, SUBFAMILY AND GENE*

1A1 1A2	2A6 2A7 2B6 2C8 2C9 2C18 2C19 2D6 2E1 2F1	3A3/4 3A5 3A7	4A9 4B1 4F2 4F3	7	11A1 11B1 11B2	17	19	21A2	27

* Key to classification: 1) The first Arabic numeral represents the family, 2) the alphabetic letter represents the subfamily, and 3) the second Arabic numeral represents the individual gene within the subfamily.

From reference: 231

TABLE 7.4 — TWO GENERAL CLASSES OF CYP ENZYMES

Families 1, 2, 3, 4

"Xenobiotic" CYP Enzymes

- Evolved from steroidogenic CYP enzymes during the period of plant-animal differentiation
- Co-evolved with transferase enzymes
- Degrade dietary toxins produced by plants
- Biotransforms drugs to permit elimination

Families 7, 11, 17, 19, 21, 27

"Steroidogenic" CYP Enzymes

- For membrane integrity of single cell organisms
- For hormonal mediators of the development of differentiated organisms
- With rigid substrate and product specificity

Data from references: 105, 115, 116, 183-185, 187

thesis of steroids and other substances necessary for the maintenance of cell wall integrity (Table 7.5). Substantial impairment in the functional integrity of the steroidogenic enzymes (eg, deficiency due to genetic mutation) is incompatible with life.

The xenobiotic CYP enzymes evolved from the steroidogenic CYP enzymes over 1 billion years ago (Table 7.4). These enzymes are located in the smooth endoplasmic reticulum of cells (Figure 7.1) and appear to have evolved during the era of plant-animal differentiation.[107, 186] The term "xenobiotic" refers to the ability of these enzymes to metabolize foreign (ie, xeno) biological substances. These enzymes allowed animals who possessed them to metabolize plant toxins before they could enter the animal's systemic circulation and cause damage. Thus, these enzymes conveyed survival advantage to the animals that possessed them.

Since drugs originally came from plants and resemble plant toxins, they can be metabolized by the same enzymes. In fact, these enzymes determine in part what substances can become drugs. If a mechanism did not exist to eliminate a substance, then that substance could not be used as a drug.

As illustrated in Figure 7.1, many drugs have a principal CYP enzyme that is responsible for the bulk, if not all, of its metabolism. In this illustration, Drug A is principally metabolized by CYP 1A2, Drug B by CYP 2D6, and Drug D by CYP 3A3/4. Drug C is an example of a drug that can be metabolized by either CYP 2D6 or 1A2.

This latter situation has caused some confusion in that it has been erroneously stated that "another enzyme could take over for an inhibited enzyme." However, these enzymes do not change their enzymatic activity or affinity for a substrate based on whether the principal enzyme is inhibited. Instead, a second enzyme comes into play when the concentration of a sub-

135

TABLE 7.5 — WHAT ARE THE FUNCTIONS OF CYP ENZYMES?

- *Steroidogenic*: conversion of consumed substances into biologically needed constituents:
  - Steroids
  - Bile acids
  - Cholesterol
  - Prostaglandin biosynthesis
- *Xenobiotic*: detoxification of consumed substances:
  - Toxins
  - Carcinogens
  - Drugs
  - Mutagens

Data from references: 105, 115, 116, 183-185, 187

FIGURE 7.1 — DRUG METABOLISM BY CYP ENZYMES

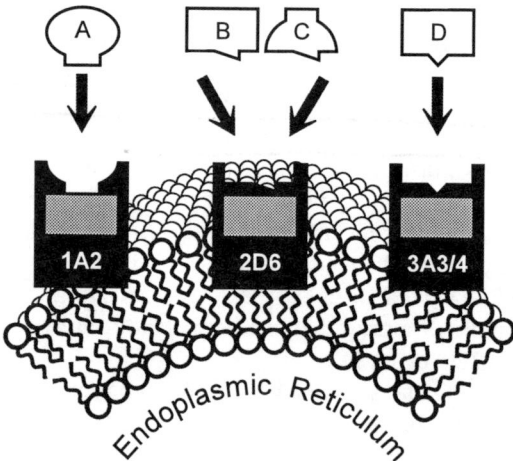

Modified from reference: 282

strate (eg, drug) such as Drug C has reached a sufficient level in the body that this pathway becomes meaningful for biotransformation and subsequent elimination.

The genetic material for these enzymes is carried in every cell in the body and expressed in multiple cells in the body. For example, CYP 2D6 is found in the brain where it is spatially linked to the dopamine uptake transporter pump.[139] However, our knowledge of the precise role of these enzymes in organs other than the liver and the bowel wall remains rudimentary.[147] In the liver and bowel wall, these enzymes are responsible for the bulk of phase I or oxidative metabolism of xenobiotics including dietary toxins, carcinogens, mutagens, and more recently, drugs. As mentioned above, their existence has permitted the development and use of medications in the treatment of patients (Table 7.5).

What Is Oxidative Metabolism?

7

Oxidative metabolism involves the conversion of a substance into a more polar species (ie, a metabolite) by the insertion or incorporation of atmospheric oxygen into the molecule (Figure 7.2). In some instances, the oxidized product is the final metabolite. In other instances, it is an intermediate metabolite and undergoes further biotransformation. CYP enzymes mediate a number of different biochemical reactions (Figure 7.3). The final result of each of these biotransformations is to produce a polar metabolite that can be eliminated in urine or feces. Often the final step is conjugation of the metabolite at a polar site with a moiety such as glucuronic acid (ie, phase II metabolism). The resulting conjugated product is water soluble and can be eliminated in the urine. This sequence from phase I to phase II metabolism and eventual elimination is illustrated in Figure 7.4.

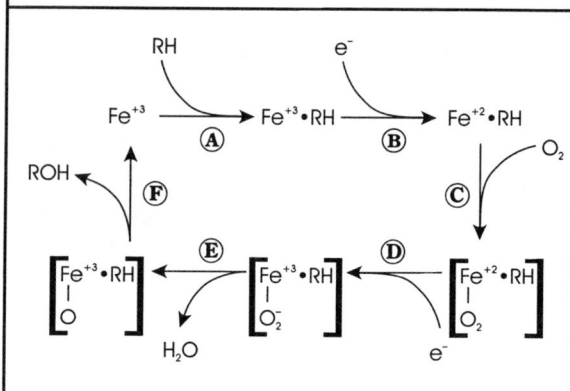

FIGURE 7.2 — CYP ENZYME REACTION CYCLE

Reference: 180

Why Do We Have Such Enzymes?

As mentioned above, the development of specific CYP enzymes had, at one time, survival value for animals by metabolizing dietary toxins before they could enter the systemic circulation. Whether these enzymes still serve such a role for man is unclear. By facilitating the biotransformation of dietary toxins, carcinogens and mutagens, these enzymes determine the total cumulative exposure to such agents in terms of both absolute concentration achieved and duration of exposure once such chemical entities are ingested.[114,117] This fact has raised the possibility that deficiency in these enzymes might be a risk factor in the development of specific diseases caused by environmental exposure to such chemicals.[53-55] For example, an active area of research is whether cigarette-induced increase in the functional activity of CYP 1A2 may explain the increased risk of some cancers in cigarette smok-

FIGURE 7.3 — DIVERSE MONOOXYGENASE ACTIVITIES OF CYP ENZYMES

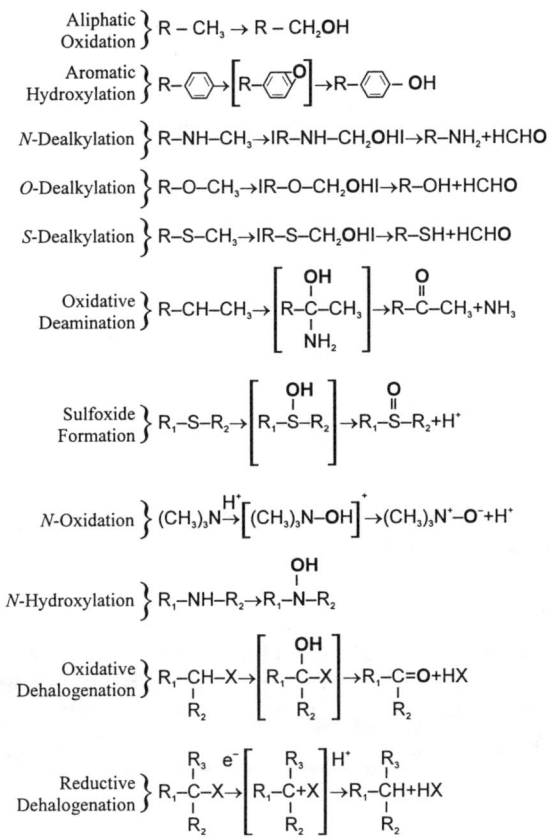

Aliphatic Oxidation } $R-CH_3 \rightarrow R-CH_2OH$

Aromatic Hydroxylation } $R-\langle\rangle \rightarrow \left[R-\langle\rangle^{O}\right] \rightarrow R-\langle\rangle-OH$

N-Dealkylation } $R-NH-CH_3 \rightarrow IR-NH-CH_2OHI \rightarrow R-NH_2+HCHO$

O-Dealkylation } $R-O-CH_3 \rightarrow IR-O-CH_2OHI \rightarrow R-OH+HCHO$

S-Dealkylation } $R-S-CH_3 \rightarrow IR-S-CH_2OHI \rightarrow R-SH+HCHO$

Oxidative Deamination } $R-CH-CH_3 \rightarrow \begin{bmatrix} OH \\ | \\ R-C-CH_3 \\ | \\ NH_2 \end{bmatrix} \rightarrow R-\overset{O}{\overset{\|}{C}}-CH_3+NH_3$

Sulfoxide Formation } $R_1-S-R_2 \rightarrow \begin{bmatrix} OH \\ | \\ R_1-S-R_2 \end{bmatrix} \rightarrow R_1-\overset{O}{\overset{\|}{S}}-R_2+H^+$

N-Oxidation } $(CH_3)_3N \overset{H^+}{\rightarrow} \left[(CH_3)_3N-OH\right]^+ \rightarrow (CH_3)_3N^+-O^-+H^+$

N-Hydroxylation } $R_1-NH-R_2 \rightarrow R_1-\overset{OH}{\overset{|}{N}}-R_2$

Oxidative Dehalogenation } $R_1-\underset{R_2}{\overset{|}{CH}}-X \rightarrow \begin{bmatrix} OH \\ | \\ R_1-C-X \\ | \\ R_2 \end{bmatrix} \rightarrow R_1-\underset{R_2}{\overset{|}{C}}=O+HX$

Reductive Dehalogenation } $R_1-\underset{R_2}{\overset{R_3}{\overset{|}{\underset{|}{C}}}}-X \overset{e^-}{\rightarrow} \begin{bmatrix} R_3 \\ | \\ R_1-C+X \\ | \\ R_2 \end{bmatrix} \overset{H^+}{\rightarrow} R_1-\underset{R_2}{\overset{R_3}{\overset{|}{\underset{|}{CH}}}}+HX$

The oxygen derived from atmospheric oxygen is denoted by boldface.

7

ers;[163,181] CYP 1A1/2 transforms some procarcinogens into carcinogens.[50,121,193] Another example is the theory that individuals genetically deficient in CYP 2D6 may

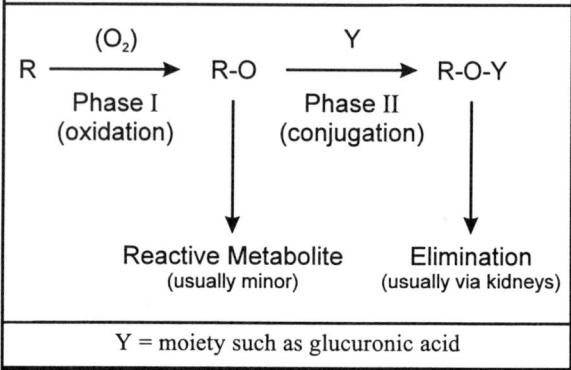

FIGURE 7.4 — PHASES OF XENOBIOTIC METABOLISM

$$R \xrightarrow{(O_2)} R\text{-}O \xrightarrow{Y} R\text{-}O\text{-}Y$$

Phase I (oxidation)　　Phase II (conjugation)

Reactive Metabolite (usually minor)　　Elimination (usually via kidneys)

Y = moiety such as glucuronic acid

have an increased risk of early-onset Parkinson's disease because they lacked this enzymatic barrier in the liver to the entry of an environmental dopamine neurotoxin such as MPTP.[17,91] The primary approach in this area of research has been to study the relative risk of different illnesses as a function of genetically determined deficiency in specific enzymes.[54]

What Is the Role of These Enzymes in Determining Response to Drug Therapy?

The functional state of these enzymes is the major determinant of the rate of biotransformation of the drug into metabolites and, hence, a major determinant of the elimination rate (ie, clearance) of specific drugs. As such, their activity determines the concentration of the drug and/or its metabolites that will be achieved in the body as a function of the dose administered (Figure 7.5). Their activity also determines the relative ratio of the administered drug to its metabolites. This

$$\frac{\text{Dosing rate}}{\text{Clearance}} \longrightarrow C_{SS} \longrightarrow \text{Response}$$

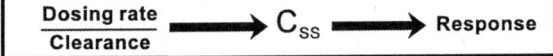

C_{SS} = Steady-state drug concentration

ratio may also be important because the metabolite(s) may be biologically active and that activity may differ in clinically important ways from that of the parent drug (eg, clomipramine and desmethylclomipramine) (see Section 3).

To put this matter in perspective, recall that the concentration(s) of the parent drug and/or its metabolites is one of the 3 variables that determines the magnitude and/or the nature of the patient's response to the drug treatment (Figure 7.6). Obviously, the drug must affect a site of action (SOA) in a specific way (ie, act as an agonist or antagonist at the SOA) to produce the desired effect. However, the magnitude of the effect is dependent on the concentration of the drug achieved at that SOA. In addition to these 2 variables, biological variance among different patients can shift the dose-response (ie, concentration-response) curve. For example, a drug such as propanolol slows heart rate by its negative chronotropic effect mediated by its mechanism of action (MOA) (ie, the blockade of β-adrenergic receptors). The higher the concentration of propanolol, the greater the degree of β-adrenergic receptor blockade, and the slower the heart rate. A patient with an underlying cardiac disease may experience a substantially greater effect at the same concentration (ie, their dose- or concentration-response

FIGURE 7.6 — RELATIONSHIP OF PHARMACODYNAMICS, PHARMACOKINETICS AND BIOLOGICAL VARIANCE IN DETERMINING OVERALL RESULT OF DRUG TREATMENT

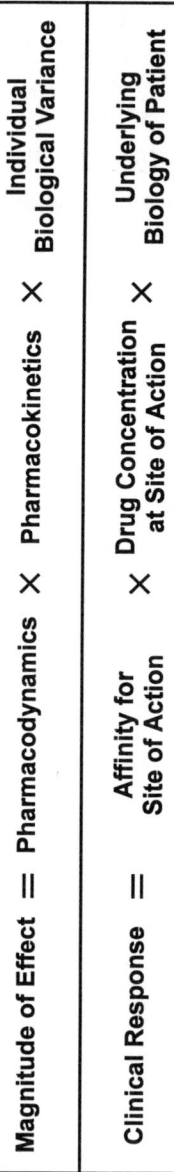

Magnitude of Effect $=$ Pharmacodynamics $\times$ Pharmacokinetics $\times$ Individual Biological Variance

Clinical Response $=$ Affinity for Site of Action $\times$ Drug Concentration at Site of Action $\times$ Underlying Biology of Patient

curve has been shifted to the left due to their underlying cardiac condition).

Since the magnitude and nature of the patient's response is concentration-dependent, the functional activity of these enzymes can make the difference between therapeutic success and failure. Such therapeutic failure may take the form of either suboptimal response or toxicity. A suboptimal response can result from the development of an inadequate concentration at the SOA due to unusually rapid clearance. Toxicity can result from the development of excessively high concentrations due to unusually slow clearance. In essence, a change in the elimination rate (ie, clearance) of a drug is the mirror image of a change in its dosing rate (Figure 7.5). Parenthetically, clearance is the amount of drug cleared per unit of time. The reason is the concentration of drug achieved in the body is directly proportional to the dosing rate and is inversely proportional to its elimination rate.

This inverse relationship is illustrated in Figure 7.5. Due to this relationship, a change in the functional activity of the enzymes mediating the biotransformation of a drug necessary for its eventual elimination typically produces an effect the opposite of what would occur with a change in the dosing rate. For example, a decrease in functional activity in the CYP enzymes will lead to a decrease in drug clearance and an increase in drug accumulation (ie, the same net effect as will occur with a dose increase). Conversely, an increase in functional activity of the enzyme would typically result in a decrease in drug accumulation (ie, a net effect similar to a dose decrease).

How Do These Enzymes Relate to Drug-Drug Interactions?

Drugs can increase or decrease the functional activity of CYP enzymes. Induction of the gene responsible for the production of the enzyme increases its rate of synthesis, thus increasing the cellular content and activity of the induced CYP enzyme.[145,206] Since induction involves protein synthesis, there is a delay in both its onset and its offset relative to starting and stopping the inducer. Therefore, the full effect may not be apparent for several weeks after the inducer has been started and the effect will take a similar period of time to fully dissipate after the inducer has been stopped and the rate of enzyme production has returned to baseline.

Drug-induced inhibition is usually competitive and occurs immediately.[278] However, the magnitude of the inhibition is a function of the concentration of the inhibitor (see Section 8). Thus, the half-life of the inhibitor will determine how long it must be administered before the full effect is achieved and, conversely, how long after its discontinuation the inhibition will persist. For this reason the full effect of fluoxetine, and particularly its long-lived active metabolite norfluoxetine, on several CYP enzymes can take several weeks to be achieved and can persist for several weeks after its discontinuation.[112,219]

How Do Such Drug-Drug Interactions Present Clinically?

There are two types of drug-drug interactions: pharmacodynamic and pharmacokinetic (Table 7.6).[224] In the former, both drugs are acting via their MOA to produce a physiological response and where the effect of one drug on its SOA amplifies or diminishes the response produced by the effect of the other drug on its SOA. For this reason, a pharmacodynamic drug interaction is likely to produce a qualitative change in the patient's response (ie, a change in the nature of the response). Examples of a qualitative change include the central serotonin syndrome that can occur when

144

TABLE 7.6 — TYPES OF DRUG INTERACTIONS	
Pharmacodynamic *MOA –* *qualitative Δ* *e.g. Seroton. Syn.*	Mechanisms of action of one drug amplifies or diminishes the effect produced by mechanisms of action of another drug.
Pharmacokinetic *quantitative Δ* *concentration*	Effect of one drug alters the pharmacokinetics of another, leading to a change in its effective concentration at its site(s) of action.
Data from reference: 213	

an SSRI and a monoamine oxidase inhibitor (MAOI) are taken together. Due to the frequently dramatic presentations of pharmacodynamic drug interactions, they are often readily identified and, hence, have received considerable attention in the medical literature.

In contrast, pharmacokinetic interactions are more likely to present as a quantitative (ie, more or less) rather than a qualitative change in the patient's response (Table 7.7). These types of interactions occur when the second drug affects the pharmacokinetics of the first drug and alters the concentration of the first drug at its SOA. In contrast to pharmacodynamic drug interactions, these interactions do not involve the addition of another effect on another SOA to the treatment equation. For this reason, a pharmacokinetic drug interaction often produces the same result as would occur with a dose change and, thus, is something that can be expected when only using the affected drug. In other words, the result is a known effect of the drug whose pharmacokinetics were altered by the addition of a second drug.

However, the effect is occurring at an unexpected dose due to the change in the drug's clearance. What the physician may not realize is that adding the sec-

TABLE 7.7 — PHARMACOKINETIC INTERACTIONS: HOW DO THEY PRESENT CLINICALLY?

- Generally quantitatively (ie, magnitude of the response) rather than qualitatively (ie, nature of the response)
- Rather than an unexpected response, such an interaction typically produces an expected response but at an unexpected dose (eg, failure to respond, adverse effect)
- This outcome is easily attributed to the patient being either "sensitive" or "resistant" to the affected drug
- May also present as an erratic response which can be dismissed as being due to noncompliance

ond drug has, in essence, changed the effective dose of the first drug by altering its clearance (Figure 7.5). Thus, the patient may appear unusually sensitive to the first drug (ie, develop a known dose-dependent adverse effect of the first drug on a dose that is usually well tolerated) or nonresponsive to the first drug (ie, failure to optimally respond to what is usually an effective dose). Thus, pharmacokinetic drug interactions may be dismissed as being due to idiosyncrasies on the part of the patient rather than being recognized for what they are.

Some examples may be useful to illustrate this concept. Risperidone is a recently marketed antipsychotic with some unique features. Figure 7.7 shows the dose-dependent nature of its antipsychotic efficacy and its risk of causing extrapyramidal adverse effects. As the dose of risperidone goes up, there is initially an increase in its antipsychotic efficacy; but somewhere between 8 to 10 mg/day, its antipsychotic efficacy either plateaus or actually begins to decrease.[169] However, the incidence and severity of extrapyramidal adverse effects continue to go up with dose increases. For these reasons, 6 mg/day is the recommended optimal dose. If a concomitantly administered drug de-

FIGURE 7.7 — DOSE-RESPONSE CURVES WITH RISPERIDONE

Antipsychotic Efficacy

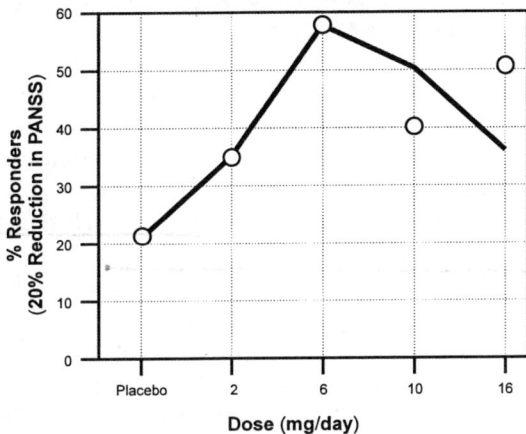

Extrapyramidal Adverse Effects

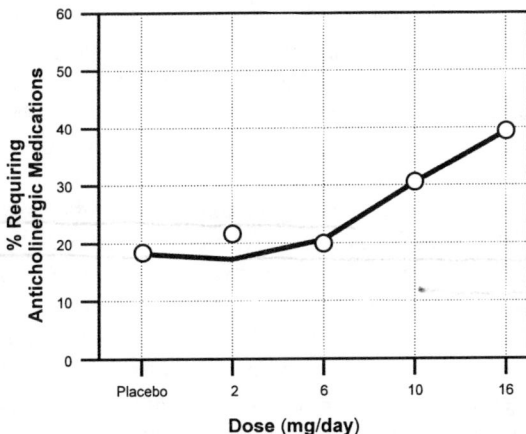

Data from reference: 169

creases the clearance of risperidone, the consequence can be the same as increasing its dose. The result will be a reduction in its efficacy and an increase in the incidence of extrapyramidal adverse effects. If the clinician does not know the dose had been effectively changed by adding the inhibitor, s/he may simply conclude that the patient is resistant to the beneficial effects and sensitive to the adverse effects of risperidone. This drug is metabolized by the CYP enzyme 2D6.

The consequences can also be more serious than loss of efficacy and increased extrapyramidal side effects. Figure 7.8 shows the seizure risk due to clozapine as a function of its daily dose. If a drug inhibits the clearance of clozapine, the consequences will be similar to increasing its dose. If the patient is on 300 mg/day and the clearance rate is reduced by 50%, this will be comparable to doubling the dose. With such a functional dose increase, the patient's risk of experiencing a seizure will go from 1.5% to 5.0% (ie, over a threefold increase in risk).

Even though such an increase in the relative risk of this potentially serious adverse effect for a given patient is substantial, it will be virtually impossible to detect in clinical practice. Since the clinician knows that some patients will have seizures even on daily doses of 300 mg/day, s/he may simply conclude that the patient is "sensitive" to this adverse effect.

To prove that such a pharmacokinetic drug interaction causes the increased risk by functionally increasing the dose would require a formal study of patients randomly assigned to clozapine with and without the inhibitor. Given the relatively infrequent nature of this adverse effect, even at doses of 600 to 900 mg/day, the study would have to involve several hundred patients to be assured of having the statistical power to detect the difference in the predicted seizure risk for the two conditions (ie, 1.5% risk versus a 5% risk). Such a study will likely never be done for ethical and

148

FIGURE 7.8 — DOSE-RESPONSE CURVES FOR SEIZURE RISK

Clozapine[1]

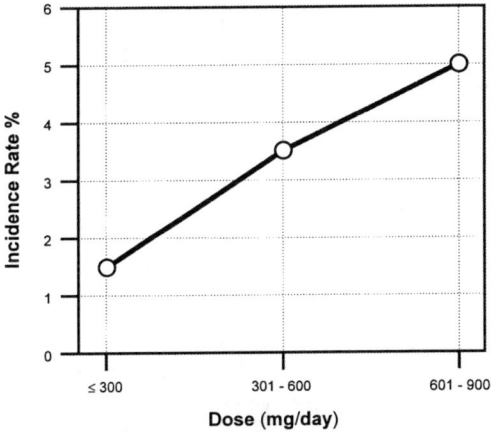

Bupropion[2]

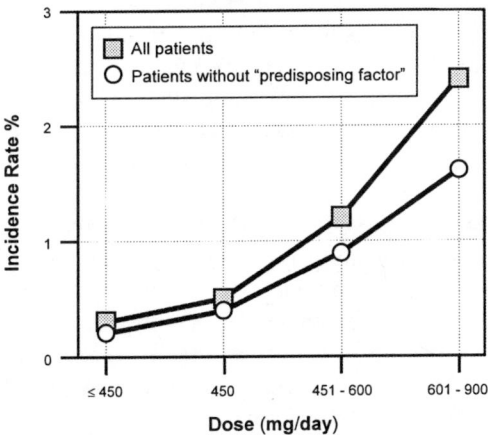

Data from references: [1]60, [2]72

economic reasons. Hence, physicians will need to make decisions based on an understanding of these principles. Of note, several CYP enzymes have been implicated in the metabolism of clozapine, including CYP 1A2, 3A3/4[208] and possibly 2D6,[255] although there is conflicting data for this CYP enzyme. Also, fluvoxamine and fluoxetine have been reported to cause moderate increases in clozapine levels,[137,300] but it is not known which enzymes they are affecting to produce this increase.

Bupropion, which is an effective antidepressant with several advantageous features,[214,220] has a dose-dependent risk of seizures (Figure 7.8). For that reason, this drug has only been marketed in the U.S.; nonetheless, it provides another good illustration of this point. Bupropion undergoes extensive biotransformation to active metabolites, but the enzymes mediating those transformations have not been established.[214] Inhibition of bupropion's clearance or the clearance of its active metabolites can increase the seizure risk just as occurs with a dose increase. Limited case data indicate that fluoxetine can produce substantial elevation of two metabolites of bupropion, although the precise mechanism for this effect has not been established.[214] Again, a large scale study of hundreds of patients would be needed to statistically test the hypothesized increased seizure risk with such a combination.

Despite the general rule being quantitative changes in response, pharmacokinetic drug interactions can sometimes produce a qualitative change in the patient's response. Two examples are provided in Table 7.8. Since qualitative changes are easier to recognize in clinical practice than are quantitative changes, these interactions are better known.

In the first type, the drug whose clearance is changed has effects on multiple SOAs in the body in a concentration-dependent manner.[221,225] Tricyclic antidepressants (TCAs) are excellent examples (Figure 7.9). At low concentrations, they block histamine and acetylcholine receptors, producing effects mediated by those actions. At therapeutic concentrations, TCAs inhibit the norepinephrine and serotonin uptake pumps believed to mediate their antidepressant efficacy. At toxic concentrations, TCAs inhibit fast sodium channels; hence, they can slow intracardiac conduction leading to serious, and even fatal, conduction disturbances. This same MOA is probably responsible for their central nervous system (CNS) toxicity (ie, delirium, seizures and coma).

If a drug inhibits the clearance of TCAs, it will have the same effect as increasing the dose of the TCA. The response to such a pharmacokinetic drug interaction may be a fatality rather than an antidepressant response.[216] That is what is meant by a change in the quality (ie, nature) of the response (eg, seizure or arrhythmia, as opposed to antidepressant efficacy) as opposed to the quantity of the response (eg, severity of dry mouth). The principal enzyme responsible for the clearance of TCAs particularly secondary amine TCAs (eg, desipramine, nortriptyline) is the CYP enzyme 2D6 which mediates the ring hydroxylation of these drugs. This conclusion is based on extensive and varied types of pharmacokinetic data.[25,40-42,45,46,48,147,195,223,262] The N-demethylation pathway, which is more prominent for tertiary amine TCAs (eg, amitriptyline, imipramine) than for secondary amine TCAs, although still not the principal route of elimination, is mediated by several CYP enzymes including CYP 1A2, 2C19 and 3A3/4.[42,46,58,161,168,192,202,256,257]

Pharmacokinetic drug interactions can also present qualitatively when the inhibition of the enzyme significantly changes the ratio of the parent drug to a metabolite which is pharmacologically active in a substantially different way than the parent drug. An example is the inhibition of the conversion of terfenadine

TABLE 7.8 — EXAMPLES OF METABOLICALLY MEDIATED PHARMACOKINETIC DRUG-DRUG INTERACTIONS AND THEIR TYPICAL CLINICAL PRESENTATIONS*

Type	Presentation	Affected Drug	Causative Drug	CYP Enzyme
Buildup of drug levels due to inhibition of clearance	Increase in incidence and/or severity of expected dose-dependent adverse effects	• Carbamazepine • Dextromethorphan • Phenytoin • Propanolol • Theophylline • Tricyclic antidepressants • Tricyclic antidepressants • Warfarin	• Erythromycin • Paroxetine • Fluoxetine • Cimetidine • Fluvoxamine • Fluoxetine • Fluvoxamine • Fluvoxamine	• 3A3/4 • 2D6 • 2C9/10 • 1A2, 3A3/4 • 1A2 • 2D6 • 1A2, 3A3/4 • 1A2
Reduction of drug levels due to induction of clearance	Loss of efficacy	• Disopyramide • Oral contraceptives • Theophylline • Propanolol • Quinidine • Theophylline • Warfarin	• Phenytoin • Carbamazepine • Phenytoin • Rifampin • Phenobarbital • Phenytoin • Secobarbital	• 3A3/4 • 3A3/4 • 1A2 • 3A3/4 • 3A3/4 • 1A2 • 1A2

Blockade of the production of an active metabolite	Loss of efficacy	• Codeine	• Paroxetine	•2D6
Increased accumulation of an unusual toxic parent drug or metabolite	Unexpected toxicity based on the usual pharmacology of the drug	• Astemizole • Terfenadine	• Ketoconazole	•3A3/4
* The above listing is in no way an exhaustive list of "causative" or "affected" drugs for either a type of interaction or for a specific CYP enzyme, but simply representative examples.				
Reference: 224				

7

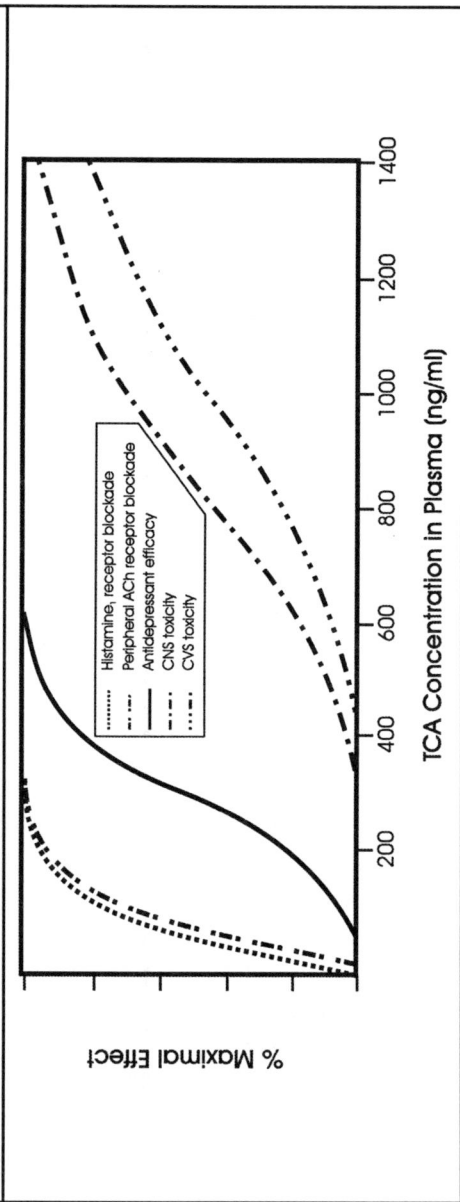

FIGURE 7.9 — MULTIPLE CONCENTRATION: RESPONSE CURVES OF TERTIARY TCAS

Legend:
- Histamine, receptor blockade
- Peripheral ACh receptor blockade
- Antidepressant efficacy
- CNS toxicity
- CVS toxicity

% Maximal Effect

TCA Concentration in Plasma (ng/ml)

Reference: 221

154

to its acid metabolite. That conversion is mediated by CYP 3A3/4 and occurs in the bowel wall and liver during the absorption of terfenadine.[295] This conversion is typically so efficient and complete that virtually all of the terfenadine is converted to its acid metabolite before entry into the systemic circulation. This metabolite is an active antihistaminic agent and is relatively devoid of effects on intracardiac conduction. Therefore, the use of terfenadine generally does not carry a risk of adverse effects on intracardiac conduction. However, terfenadine itself does inhibit intracardiac conduction and can cause arrhythmias.[258] If the conversion of terfenadine to its acid metabolite is substantially blocked during absorption, then terfenadine will enter the systemic circulation. If its concentrations are sufficiently high, cardiac arrhythmias can result. Thus, coadministration of terfenadine with a potent inhibitor of CYP 3A3/4 can have serious, and even life-threatening, adverse consequences.[297] Ketoconazole related antifungal agents and several macrolide antibiotics (eg, erythromycin) can substantially inhibit this enzyme.[29,126,127,279] Fluvoxamine, norfluoxetine and the non-SSRI antidepressant, nefazodone, also inhibit this enzyme, but are substantially less potent than ketoconazole in this regard.[144,276]

Where Are We Going With This Knowledge?

Two sets of knowledge are now being developed as illustrated in Figure 7.10. The first is which drugs affect which CYP enzymes, either by induction or inhibition. The second is which drugs are metabolized by a specific CYP enzyme (Table 7.9). With these two sets of knowledge, we can determine whether the coadministration of one drug is likely to affect the biotransformation of another drug. We can also determine whether the second drug is likely to alter the over-

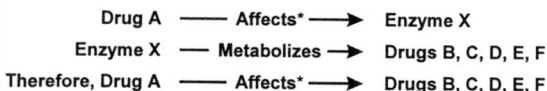

all clearance (ie, elimination rate) of the first drug and hence its accumulation on a given dose and whether the second drug is likely to affect the relative ratio of specific metabolites to the parent drug by inducing or inhibiting a specific biotransformation pathway. In addition to the examples already given, the coadministration of an inhibitor or an inducer might increase the production of what is normally a minor metabolite to a substantial extent. This metabolite may mediate clinically important effects. For example, the increased risk of hepatoxicity when valproate is coadministered with another anticonvulsant (ie, carbamazepine or phenytoin) may have been due to the increased production of the 4-ene metabolite of valproate via the induction of the CYP enzyme that mediates the conversion.[169]

In the past, this type of pharmacokinetic drug interaction could not be anticipated, but had to occur and then be identified clinically after the fact. Early pharmacokinetic drug interaction studies were done mainly on the basis of what drugs were likely to be used together rather than because there was a substantial reason to suspect a clinically meaningful drug-drug interaction. Physicians had to remember these types of interactions without having any organizing principles to aid them.

156

Due to improved knowledge of CYP enzymes, this situation has substantially changed. Now studies can be done by deductive reasoning using the 3 sets of information illustrated in Figure 7.10. From a research standpoint, this knowledge will permit the anticipation of clinically meaningful interactions which can then be confirmed by focused formal pharmacokinetic drug interactions studies done under clinically relevant conditions. From a clinical standpoint, this knowledge will allow physicians to anticipate such an interaction and make appropriate drug and dose selections to avoid undesired consequences.

This knowledge is also being used to determine what drugs to develop. New candidate drugs are now tested for how they are metabolized and whether they affect specific CYP enzymes. A new candidate drug may not be developed based on the results of such tests if it is principally metabolized by a CYP enzyme that is inducible or inhibited by many commonly used drugs or is genetically deficient in a sizable percentage of the population (Table 7.10). Also, a new drug may not be developed if it induces or inhibits CYP enzymes responsible for the metabolism of many other drugs.

If the unique efficacy of the new drug outweighs these considerations, then the information about how it is metabolized and its affects on the CYP enzymes will be used to help guide its safe and effective use in clinical practice. For example, this information can be entered into a readily accessible computer database; the physician can enter the patient's current treatment into a computer and the new drug which is going to be added to the regimen. Using such an information system, the physician can quickly determine:

- Whether an interaction is likely
- The nature of the interaction, including its potential seriousness
- What adjustment should be made in terms of dosage

TABLE 7.9—DRUGS METABOLIZED
BY CYP ENZYMES*

CYP 1A2

Antidepressants—amitriptyline, clomipramine, imipramine
Antipsychotics—clozapine
β-*Blockers*—propanolol
Miscellaneous—caffeine, paracetamol, theophylline,
R-warfarin

CYP 2C9/10

phenytoin, S-warfarin, tolbutamide

CYP 2C19

Antidepressants—citalopram, clomipramine, imipramine
Barbiturates—hexobarbital, mephobarbital, S-mephenytoin
Benzodiazepines—diazepam
β-*Blockers*—propranolol

CYP 2D6

Antiarrhythmics—encainide, flecainide, mexiletine,
propafenone
Antipsychotics—haloperidol, perphenazine, risperidone,
thioridazine
β-*Blockers*—alprenolol, bufarolol, metoprolol, propranolol,
timolol
Miscellaneous—debrisoquin, 4-hydroamphetamine,
perhexiline, phenformin, sparteine
Opiates—codeine, dextromethorphan, ethylmorphine
SSRIs—fluoxetine, N-desmethylcitalopram, paroxetine
TCAs—amitriptyline, clomipramine, desipramine,
imipramine, N-desmethylclomipramine, clomipramine,
nortriptyline, trimipramine
Other Antidepressants—venlafaxine, the mCPP metabolite of
nefazodone and trazodone

CYP 3A3/4

Analgesics—acetaminophen, alfentanil, codeine,
dextromethorphan
Antiarrhythmics—amiodarone, disopyramide, lidocaine,
propafenone, quinidine
Anticonvulsants—carbamazepine, ethosuximde

Antidepressants—amitriptyline, clomipramine, imipramine, nefazodone, sertraline, *O*-desmethylvenlafaxine

Antiestrogens—docetaxel, paclitaxel, tamoxifen

Antihistamines—astemizole, loratadine, terfenadine

Antipsychotics—clozapine

Benzodiazepines—alprazolam, clonazepam, diazepam, midazolam, triazolam

Calcium Channel Blockers—diltiazem, felodipine, nicardipine, nifedipine, niludipine, minodipine, nisoldipine, nitrendipine, verapamil

Immunosuppressants—cyclosporine, tacrolimus (FK506—macrolide)

Local Anesthetics—cocaine, lidocaine

Macrolide Antibiotics—clarithromycin, erythromycin, triacetyloleandomycin

Steroids—androstendione, cortisol, dihydroepiandrosterone 3-sulfate, dexamethasone, estradiol, ethinylestradiol, progesterone, testosterone

Miscellaneous—benzphetamine, cisapride, dapsone, lovastatin, omeprazole (sulfonation)

---

* Major pathway for elimination of tricylcic antidepressants is ring hydroxylation; *N*-desmethylation, a minor pathway, is mediated by several CYP enzymes.

NOTE: Tables such as this are limited by our current knowledge. The CYP enzyme(s) responsible for biotransformation has been determined for only approximately 20% of marketed drugs. Many drugs were developed before the necessary knowledge and technology existed. Hence, these lists are first attempts but will become more comprehensive as we backfill our knowledge base. Also note that some drugs are listed under more than one CYP enzyme since different enzymes mediate either the same or different metabolic pathways. That does not necessarily mean that each of these enzymes contribute equally to the elimination of the drug. One enzyme may be principally responsible based on the substrate affinity and the capacity and abundance of the enzyme.

Adapted from references: 39, 119, 144

TABLE 7.10 — GENETICALLY DETERMINED CYP ENZYME DEFICIENCY			
CYP	Orientals	Blacks	Whites
2C19	20%	Not known	3%
2D6	1%	4%	8%
Data from references: 104, 152			

- What drug can be substituted for the proposed new drug to avoid the interaction

Patients can also be genotyped and phenotyped for specific CYP enzyme activity, and that information can also be entered into the computer database along with their current treatment regimen and any proposed changes. This additional information will further increase the accuracy of the predictions and recommendations. Obviously, the development of this knowledge has substantial implications for improving patient care in terms of safety, tolerability and efficacy. Those implications extend well beyond any single class of medications, but nonetheless, have specific implications now for the SSRI class of antidepressants as discussed in Section 8.

8

How Does This Knowledge Relate to the Clinical Use of SSRIs?

The effect of specific serotonin selective reuptake inhibitors (SSRIs) on specific cytochrome P450 (CYP) enzymes has been the major distinguishing factor among these drugs and is clinically important for three reasons:

- First, these medications are extensively used in the general population.
- Second, many physicians use these antidepressants, preferentially in the elderly and medically-ill with major depression due to their generally benign safety profile (Table 8.1).
- Third, their long-term maintenance use is growing due to the recognition that major depression is frequently a recurring illness, and prophylactic treatment with an antidepressant can decrease the risk of recurrent episodes. During such prophylactic treatment, the patient may develop an intercurrent illness (eg, hypertension) and require the addition of another medication.

For all of these reasons, there is a substantial likelihood that the patient who is taking an SSRI will be treated with another medication and hence will be at potential risk for a drug-drug interaction.

Consistent with these observations, several recent surveys have shown that many patients being treated with an antidepressant were also taking other medications and, hence, had the potential to experience a drug-drug interaction (Table 8.2).

TABLE 8.1 — PREVALENCE OF MAJOR DEPRESSION IN SPECIFIC MEDICALLY ILL POPULATIONS

Medical Illness	Prevalence
Terminal solid tumors	25% to 38%
Stroke	27% to 35%
Renal disease	5% to 22%
Chronic pain	35% to > 50%
Epilepsy	20% to 30%
Parkinson's disease	30% to 50%
Myocardial infarction	20%
Diabetes mellitus	10%
Data from references: 83, 241, 248	

TABLE 8.2 — CONCOMITANT USE OF AN ANTIDEPRESSANT WITH OTHER MEDICATIONS IN DIFFERENT PATIENT POPULATIONS

Source	Population	Three or more
Holm et al, 1990[1]	Outpatients in general primary care practice	30%
Preskorn et al, 1995[2]	Patients in medical school outpatient psychiatric clinic	45%
Coulehan et al, 1990[3]	Outpatients with depressive symptoms in a medical school primary care clinic	60%
Wolf et al, 1995[4]	"Chronic" outpatients in a Veterans Administration psychiatric clinic	60%
References: [1]125, [2]212, [3]62, [4]289		

As discussed in Section 3, one of the goals in the rational development of the SSRIs was to reduce the likelihood of pharmacodynamic drug interactions. Originally, the goal was to avoid the multiple types of pharmacodynamic drug interactions that can occur when using tricyclic antidepressants (TCAs) in combination with other drugs due to the multiple mechanisms of action (MOAs) of TCAs. While SSRIs were developed to avoid this problem, they were developed before we had the ability to screen for effects on the CYP enzymes. This fact explains why there are so many differences among SSRIs with regard to their effects on these enzymes. In essence, the action of some of the SSRIs on these enzymes is analogous to the effect of TCAs on fast sodium channels: these effects are unintended and unnecessary relative to the desired goal of treating major depression. Instead of adding to their efficacy, the inhibition of these enzymes produces the undesired risk of causing pharmacokinetic drug interactions. This section will focus on the differential effects of SSRIs on specific CYP enzymes and their potential for causing such interactions.

A separate issue is whether the inhibition of these enzymes has any long-term consequences (Table 8.3). This issue, while only theoretical now, is potentially important since patients may remain on SSRIs for years to prevent recurrent depressive episodes. For example, prophylactic treatment with fluoxetine and paroxetine essentially converts the patient into a phenocopy of genetic deficiency of the CYP enzyme 2D6 (Table 8.4). Due to the widespread use of SSRIs for maintenance treatment, a relatively large segment of the population is being converted into phenocopies of CYP 2D6 deficiency. Obviously, this enzyme is not essential to life given the rather widespread (approximately 7%) incidence of its deficiency in Caucasians. However, it will be important to know whether functional activity of this enzyme is a risk factor for the development of

TABLE 8.3 — CAN INHIBITION OF CYP ENZYMES HAVE OTHER CONSEQUENCES?
• Can be used intentionally to delay or change the metabolism of another drug
• Since CYP enzymes such as CYP 2D6 are found extrahepatically, such inhibition may have other consequences (either desirable or undesirable) on organ function other than the liver
• Are there any long-term consequences of altering the clearance rate of the natural substrates for such an enzyme?

chronic illnesses.[3,53,55,61,88,138,231] This issue requires specific study as discussed in Section 7.

Myths Concerning SSRIs and CYP Enzymes

Perhaps as a result of the intense competition among these drugs, there has been a considerable amount of disinformation about the issue of CYP enzymes and SSRIs. A number of myths have arisen that may cause confusion (Table 8.5). Many of these myths involve the effects of these drugs on the enzyme CYP 2D6, probably because this enzyme was the first one shown to be substantially inhibited by some SSRIs. One myth is that the inhibition of these enzymes, particularly CYP 2D6, is a class issue with SSRIs. A subset of this myth is that only the *in vitro* potency of these drugs needs to be compared to determine their relative clinical effects without regard to the different concentration of different SSRIs achieved under clinically relevant conditions. A second myth is that the inhibition of these enzymes affects only one or perhaps a couple of drugs. A third myth is that all the drugs affected by the inhibition of a specific CYP enzyme are known.

TABLE 8.4 — SOME SSRIs LACK SELECTIVITY WITH REGARD TO EFFECTS ON SEROTONIN UPTAKE VERSUS CYP 2D6

SSRI	Usually Effective, Antidepressant Dose (mg/day)[1]	Plasma Level (ng/ml)[1]	Serotonin Uptake[1]	CYP 2D6[2]
Citalopram	40	≈ 85	≈ 60%	≈ 15%
Fluoxetine	20	≈ 200	≈ 80%	≈ 85%
Fluvoxamine	150	≈ 100	≈70%	< 15%
Paroxetine	20	≈ 40	≈ 80%	≈ 85%
Sertraline	50	≈ 25	≈ 80%	≈ 15%

[1]See Table 3.7.
[2]See Table 8.9.

TABLE 8.5 — COMMON MYTHS ABOUT CYP ENZYMES AND SSRIS

- The effect is a class issue in which all drugs affect "the enzyme" to the same extent.
- Effects on CYP 2D6 are responsible for all the effects of all the SSRIs.
- Other CYP enzymes will "take over" for the inhibited enzyme.
- The clinical significance is limited to a few drugs.

In this section, we will address these myths by reviewing our current knowledge of the effects of the SSRIs on specific CYP enzymes. We will first review how this information has been developed so that the reader can understand, and even anticipate, future developments in our knowledge about the relative effects of drugs, SSRIs and others, on these enzymes. While this book is on SSRIs, the issue of drugs affecting CYP enzymes is not restricted to this class. They are merely examples of this phenomenon and thus serve to illustrate a larger point.

How Do We Determine the Effects of Specific Drugs on Specific CYP Enzymes?

Our knowledge in this area comes from both *in vitro* and *in vivo* studies (Table 8.6). *In vitro* studies can be used to determine how potent a specific drug is as an inhibitor of a specific CYP enzyme. *In vivo* studies are done to determine whether the interaction occurs and to what extent under clinically relevant conditions. A brief description of the two different approaches follows as a frame of reference for the remainder of this section.

TABLE 8.6 — DRUG-INDUCED INHIBITION OF CYP ENZYMES

- Typically competitive inhibition
- Delays clearance of other substances causing increased and prolonged accumulation (eg, pharmacokinetic interactions)
- Can be studied both *in vitro* and *in vivo* — Questions that can be answered by these two types of studies:
  - *In vitro*:
    - Does a drug have the potential to inhibit a specific CYP enzyme?
    - If a pharmacokinetic interaction has been observed, an effect on what CYP enzyme mediates the interaction?
  - *In vivo*:
    - Does an interaction occur under clinically relevant dosing conditions?

■ *In Vitro* Studies

Several different techniques can be used in these studies, including the use of:

- Purified enzyme
- Liver slices
- Human hepatic microsome preparations
- Cells transvected with a specific human CYP gene

These techniques can be used to determine whether a specific human CYP enzyme is responsible for the metabolism of specific drugs and whether specific drugs are capable of altering the functional activity of a specific human CYP enzyme. Presently, the most common approach employs microsome preparations. After an appropriate series of samples have been prepared, a substrate (eg, a drug known to be metabolized by that enzyme) for the enzyme is added in a predetermined concentration. Then, the potential inhibitor is added in varying concentrations to determine its potency for blocking the enzyme-mediated biotransformation of the substrate. This approach is analogous to determining the binding affinity of a drug to a specific neuroreceptor (see Section 3). The results of such *in vitro* studies for the various SSRIs for 3 important CYP enzymes are shown in Table 8.7.

While the *in vitro* potency is an important determinant of the potential for a drug to produce an effect, it is not the sole determinant. Obviously, the drug must reach a sufficient concentration at the site of action (SOA) (which is the CYP enzyme in this instance) to produce sufficient inhibition of the enzyme to be clinically meaningful. In the case of a pharmacokinetic interaction, this means the inhibition of the enzyme must be sufficient to cause a clinically meaningful change (either an increase or decrease depending on the interaction in question) in the plasma and tissue concentration of a concomitantly administered drug which is dependent on that CYP enzyme for its clearance. There is no simple way to determine whether the degree of inhibition that will be achieved by two drugs will be the same or different based solely on their relative *in vitro* potency for inhibiting an enzyme. Instead, the relative concentrations of the drugs under clinically relevant conditions must be taken into account. Moreover, it is not the plasma drug concentration that is critical but rather the concentration at the enzyme.

Mathematical modeling can be done to estimate the degree of enzyme inhibition that will be produced by a given drug under clinically relevant conditions based on a knowledge of 3 factors:

- *In vitro* inhibition constant of the drug for that specific enzyme
- Plasma concentration of the drug that occurs under those conditions

- Plasma:hepatic partition coefficient for that drug under those conditions

Many readers may not be interested in more details concerning such modeling work beyond knowing that it exists and what its implications are. For those who are interested in more details, see Section 10, *Appendix*.

The important application of such modeling is that it can help to determine whether a specific pharmacokinetic interaction is likely to occur to a clinically meaningful extent when that drug is coprescribed with a drug that is dependent on that enzyme for its elimination. This approach can help to rationally guide research to focus on the most critical pharmacokinetic studies (ie, those which are likely to reveal an important interaction). This is a significant advance over the previous approach where drugs were studied simply because they had a higher likelihood of being coprescribed together or because interactions had been described with other drugs in a "class" such as "antidepressants" which includes vastly different drugs such as TCAs, SSRIs and monoamine oxidase inhibitors (MAOIs).

Although such modeling work is an important screening tool to focus research on highly likely interactions, a definitive answer as to whether a drug will inhibit a CYP enzyme to a sufficient extent to produce a clinically meaningful drug-drug interaction requires formal *in vivo* pharmacokinetic interaction studies done under clinically relevant dosing conditions. In such studies, the degree of enzyme inhibition is typically measured by changes in the pharmacokinetics of a drug dependent on a specific CYP enzyme for its clearance in the absence, and then in the presence, of the potential inhibitor.

8

TABLE 8.7 — THE RELATIVE POTENCY* OF FIVE DIFFERENT SSRIS AND THEIR METABOLITES FOR INHIBITING THE FUNCTIONAL INTEGRITY OF THREE CYP ENZYMES 1A2, 2D6 AND 3A3/4 BASED ON *IN VITRO* STUDIES USING HUMAN HEPATIC MICROSOMES

Study	Citalopram/desmethylcitalopram	Fluoxetine/Norfluoxetine	Fluovoxamine	Paroxetine/M2	Sertraline/desmethylsertraline
		CYP 1A2			
Brosen et al[1]	>100/>100	>100/>100	0.2	45/NA	70/NA
Rasmussen et al[2]	>100/>100	>100/>100	0.2	50	>100
von Moltke et al[3]	NA	4.4/5.9	0.24	5.5	8.8/9.5
		CYP 2D6			
Crewe et al[4]	5.1	0.60/0.45	8.2	0.15/0.50	0.70/NA
Skjelbo et al[5]	19/1.3	0.92/0.33	3.9	0.36/NA	—
Von Moltke et al[6†]	—	3.0/3.5	16.6	2.0/NA	22.7/16.9
Otton et al[7]	—	0.17/0.19	—	—	1.5/NA

			CYP 3A3/4[†]		
Otton et al[8]	—	0.15/NA	—	0.065/NA	1.2/NA
Von Moltke et al[9]	—	83.3/11.1	10	39/NA	23.8/20.4
Rasmussen et al[2]	>100/ >100	60/19	40	70	90

* *In vitro* potency = K_i = inhibition constant; the smaller the value, the greater the potency on a molar basis.

[†] K_i values for comparison: quinidine = 626; ketoconazole = 0.05[10]

NA = Not applicable

References: [1]47, [2]235, [3]299, [4]464, [5]256, [6]278, [7]196, [8]194, [9]279, [10]276

8

■ *In Vivo* Studies

The general design for a formal *in vivo* pharmaco-kinetic study is given in Figure 8.1. The essence of these studies is to determine whether the coadministration of the potential inhibitor or inducer alters the clearance of a concomitantly administered drug that is a model substrate for the enzyme in question. Ideally, such studies use a model substrate which is a drug that is solely metabolized by one CYP enzyme and does not itself alter this enzyme's activity (ie, no auto-induction or autoinhibition) over the clinically relevant concentration range.

The first step is to give the model substrate to normal volunteers to determine its rate of biotransformation and elimination (ie, its clearance) in the absence of the potential inhibitor or inducer. Two different dosing strategies have been used with regard to the administration of the model substrate.

In the single dose approach, the clearance of the model substrate in a volunteer is quantitated after a single dose in the absence and presence of the potential inhibitor or inducer. The latter is usually dosed to steady-state prior to the single-dose rechallenge of the model substrate. In the multiple dose approach, the model substrate is administered to the volunteer on a daily basis for a sufficiently long enough interval to ensure that its steady-state has been achieved. The potential inhibitor or inducer is then added to the regimen at a clinically relevant dose and administered sufficiently long enough to ensure it has also reached steady-state conditions. The clearance of the model substrate is measured before and after the addition of the potential inhibitor or inducer. The multiple dose approach is more rigorous and more expensive, and more closely mimics clinical practice than does the single dose approach.

In both approaches, the potential inhibitor or inducer is administered on a multiple dose basis in an

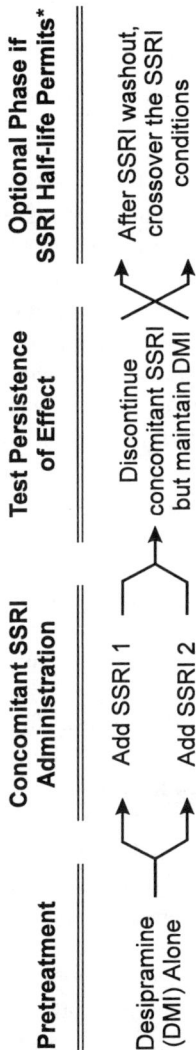

FIGURE 8.1 — DESIGN OF PHARMACOKINETIC INTERACTION STUDIES USING SSRIS AS AN EXAMPLE

Pretreatment

Desipramine (DMI) Alone

Concomitant SSRI Administration

Add SSRI 1

Add SSRI 2

Test Persistence of Effect

Discontinue concomitant SSRI but maintain DMI

Optional Phase if SSRI Half-life Permits*

After SSRI washout, crossover the SSRI conditions

* Generally impractical with fluoxetine due to the protracted interval needed for washout of that SSRI and its effect on CYP enzymes.

8

173

analogous way to how it would be given in clinical practice. Changes in the plasma levels and clearance of the model substrate quantitatively reflect the degree of enzyme inhibition or induction produced by the potential inhibitor or inducer respectively under clinically relevant conditions.

In the past, *in vitro* and *in vivo* studies have been done in a nonsystematic, nonsequential fashion. For example, *in vivo* studies might be done before *in vitro* studies or, even though an *in vitro* or *in vivo* study might be positive, the other type of study might not be done. An *in vitro* study might show that a specific drug has an inhibition potency such that one would expect that the effect could occur under clinically relevant conditions, but the confirmatory *in vivo* studies might not be done. For these reasons, there are gaps in our current knowledge, but they are in the process of being filled.

The trend now is for these studies to be done using a more sequential approach. For efficiency, *in vitro* studies are done first to screen for potentially meaningful effects of an investigational drug on a specific CYP enzyme. Those studies determine the *in vitro* potency of the investigational drug for inhibiting or inducing the enzyme. This information, coupled with a knowledge of what concentration of the investigational drug is achieved under clinically relevant conditions, can be used to predict whether this drug is likely to produce meaningful inhibition or induction of the enzyme under clinically relevant conditions. Then, *in vivo* studies are done to confirm cases where it is likely a pharmacokinetic drug interaction will occur under such conditions. The *in vivo* follow-up studies are done with drugs (ie, model substrates) that can serve as *in vivo* probes to quantify the functional activity of the enzyme before and after the coadministration of the investigational drug (ie, the potential inhibitor or inducer). The results of the *in vivo* studies can also be used to predict whether other drugs that are substrates for that specific CYP enzyme will be affected when they are coadministered with the investigational drug under clinically relevant conditions.

Obviously, this approach is not restricted to SSRIs but can be used with any drug suspected of affecting a specific CYP enzyme. Research with SSRIs has simply been pioneering work in this area and has documented that several SSRIs are capable of inhibiting one or more CYP enzyme to a clinically meaningful extent under clinically relevant conditions.

Beyond this systematic approach to detecting potential pharmacokinetic drug interactions, spontaneous observation in clinical practice can lead to case reports. These reports can serve the useful purpose of guiding formal research, particularly when there is *in vitro* data that also supports the probability of an interaction under clinically relevant conditions. Nonetheless, case reports are only suggestive and not definitive and clearly cannot be equated with the results from formal pharmacokinetic studies due to the limited amount of data and the typical absence of adequate controls. For example, there is often no control for compliance in such case reports and the interpretation is highly dependent on the validity of the first sample obtained, which is typically done on an outpatient basis.

8

What Do We Know About the Effects of Specific SSRIs on Specific CYP Enzymes?

The results from the studies that have been done on 5 major xenobiotic CYP enzymes (ie, CYP 1A2, 2C9/10, 2C19, 2D6 and 3A3/4) follows and is also summarized in 2 tables. Table 8.8 presents a composite summary based on the available formal *in vitro* and *in vivo* studies. As can be seen from the table, there is

TABLE 8.8 — EFFECTS OF SPECIFIC SSRIs ON SPECIFIC CYP ENZYMES AT THEIR RESPECTIVE, USUALLY EFFECTIVE, ANTIDEPRESSANT DOSE*

Enzyme	Citalopram	Fluoxetine	Fluvoxamine	Paroxetine	Sertraline
CYP 1A2	Unlikely[1]	Unlikely[1]	Substantial[1,2]	Unlikely[1]	Unlikely[1]
CYP 2C9/10	?	?[3]	?	NCS[2]	NCS[2]
CYP 2C19	?	Moderate[2]	Substantial[2]	?	NCS[2]
CYP 2D6	Mild[1]	Substantial[1,2]	NCS[1,2]	Substantial[1,2]	Mild[1,2]
CYP 3A3/4	?	Mild[1,2]	Moderate[1,2]	Unlikely[1,2]	Unlikely[1,2,4]

? = absence of or contradictory *in vitro* or *in vivo* data available for this SSRI

Unlikely = based on *in vitro* studies, unlikely to have a clinically meaningful effect

NCS = not clinically significant in most situations = < 20% change†

Mild = 20% to 50% change†

Moderate = 50% to 150% change†

Substantial = > 150% change†

† Change in the area under the curve (AUC) of the plasma level-time curve of a substrate (ie, concomitantly administered drug) dependent on that CYP enzyme for its clearance.

* Table is a summary of the results presented in Tables 8.7, 8.9, 8.11, and 10.1, and data reviewed in the text. Hence, it is based on effects observed or predicted based on the concentration of these drugs that would be usually produced by their usually effective, antidepressant dose. Since the inhibition of these enzymes is concentration-dependent, the magnitude of the effect will be higher on average at higher doses particularly for SSRIs with nonlinear pharmacokinetics (see Table 6.2).

[1] Predicted based on *in vitro* inhibitory rate constants and on knowledge about clinically relevant plasma drug levels (for details about predictive modelling, see Section 10, *Appendix*).

[2] Based on the following *in vivo* data: A large number of well documented case reports principally involving theophylline for fluvoxamine's effect on CYP 1A2 and formal *in vivo* studies is summarized in Table 8.9 for effects on CYP 2D6 and Table 8.11 for effects on CYP 2C9/10, 2C19, and 3A3/4. Relative to CYP 3A3/4, data with paroxetine and sertraline are limited to carbamezepine rather than a more model substrate such as alprazolam.

[3] Studies with tolbutamide and warfarin suggest no effects, but 23 cases with adequate data with phenytoin suggest a substantial effect of fluoxetine on CYP 2C9/10. The reasons for the discrepancy in these results are not clear.

[4] The designation, "unlikely," is further supported by the linear pharmacokinetics of sertraline over its full dosing range (ie, 50 to 200 mg/day) since sertraline is demethylated by CYP 3A3/4 (see Section 6).

8

a variable amount of data with regard to both a specific enzyme and the effects of a specific SSRI. Data relative to a specific CYP enzyme may be available for some, but not all, SSRIs. Data may come solely from either *in vitro* or *in vivo* studies and sometimes data from both types of studies are available, which is the ideal situation. Occasionally, only suggestive case reports are available, either alone or combined with *in vitro* studies. Again, data based on case reports, particularly when limited to a small number of patients, must be interpreted in a cautious manner and not equated with results from formal, rigorous studies. Table 8.7 summarizes the results of the *in vitro* studies that have been done with the SSRIs relative to three specific enzymes: CYP 1A2, 2D6 and 3A3/4. Tables 8.9 and 8.11 summarize the *in vivo* studies.

■ **CYP 1A2**

The data regarding the differential effects of SSRIs on CYP 1A2 come principally from 2 *in vitro* studies (Table 8.7). Brosen et al and Rasmussen et al have shown that fluvoxamine has an inhibitory rate constant for this enzyme such that it is likely to cause clinically meaningful inhibition under antidepressant treatment conditions (Table 8.7). Consistent with these *in vitro* findings, there is evidence that fluvoxamine inhibits the clearance of drugs dependent on this enzyme for biotransformation prior to elimination. While the rate-limiting step for the elimination of all TCAs is ring hydroxylation mediated by CYP 2D6,[14,15,25,38,40-42,45,46,48,67,109,161,171,192,195,205,262] the tertiary amine TCAs are demethylated by several CYP enzymes including CYP 1A2, 3A3/4 and possibly 2C19. [19,38,41,42,46,58,118,161,168,192,202,247,256,257,262] Concomitant administration of fluvoxamine inhibits such demethylation and produces higher than usual concentrations of the parent drug (ie, tertiary amine TCAs such as clomipramine)

#	Study	Reference	Drug	Dose	Substrate	Result
1	Gram et al, 1993	110	Citalopram	40 mg/d	IMI/DMI	↑ 47%
2	Bergstrom et al, 1992	24	Fluoxetine	60 mg/d (7 days)	DMI	↑ 640%
3	Preskorn et al, 1994	219	Fluoxetine	20 mg/d (3 wks)	DMI	↑ 380%
4	Spina et al, 1993	263	Fluvoxamine	100 mg/d	IMI/DMI	↑ 14%
5	Albers et al, 1995	4	Paroxetine	30 mg/d	IMI/DMI	↑ 327%
6	Alderman et al, 1996	5	Paroxetine	20 mg/d	DMI	↑ 421%
7	Brosen et al, 1993	41	Paroxetine	20 mg/d	DMI	↑ 364%
8	Jann et al, 1996	136	Sertraline	50 mg/d	IMI	0%
9	Preskorn et al, 1994	219	Sertraline	50 mg/d	DMI	↑ 23%
10	Alderman et al, 1996	5	Sertraline	50 mg/d	DMI	↑ 37%
11	Sproule et al, 1995	264	Sertraline	108 mg/d	Dextromethorpan	↑ 5%
12	Zussman et al, 1994	298	Sertraline	150 mg/d	DMI	↑ 54%
13	Kurtz et al, 1994	153	Sertraline	150 mg/d	DMI	↑ 70%

TABLE 8.9 — *IN VIVO* STUDIES OF EFFECTS OF DIFFERENT SSRIS ON CYP 2D6 FUNCTION

8

**TABLE 8.10 — RELATIVE POTENCY OF THE
ENANTIOMERS OF FLUOXETINE AND
NORFLUOXETINE FOR INHIBITING
THE CYP ENZYME 2D6**

Enantiomer	Kinetic inhibitory constant K_i (μm)[1]
S-fluoxetine	0.22
R-fluoxetine	1.38
S-norfluoxetine	0.31
R-norfluoxetine	1.48
S/R ratio for fluoxetine and norfluoxetine = 2.2[2]	
S/R ratio = ratio of plasma levels of the 2 enantiomer under steady-state conditions when the racemic mixture is being taken.	
Data from references: [1]267, [2]272	

relative to their demethylated metabolite (ie, a secondary amine TCA such as desmethylclomipramine) (see Section 3).[18,27,28,118] Fluvoxamine can also produce clinically significant elevations of theophylline and clozapine, drugs dependent on CYP 1A2 for their metabolism.[137,260,270,274]

Based on the results from the Brosen et al and Rasmussen et al *in vitro* studies, the other SSRIs would not be expected to inhibit CYP 1A2 to any meaningful extent under clinically relevant conditions (Table 8.7). While there are no formal *in vivo* studies, there is indirect *in vivo* evidence to support this conclusion. Although concomitant administration of fluvoxamine produces a substantial increase in warfarin plasma levels (+ 65%),[22] this effect does not occur with fluoxetine, paroxetine or sertraline.[16,245,287]

Warfarin is a racemic mixture. *S*-warfarin is metabolized by CYP 2C9/10 and is the active enantiomer in terms of anticoagulant effect.[149,162,238] The inactive *R*-warfarin enantiomer is metabolized by CYP 1A2 but can inhibit CYP 2C9/10 and thus produce an accumulation of the active *S*-warfarin enantiomer. The fact that fluvoxamine produces a buildup of warfarin plasma levels is compatible with the inhibition of CYP 1A2 and a resultant buildup of *R*-warfarin plasma levels which in turn inhibit CYP 2C9/10, resulting in a buildup of *S*-warfarin plasma levels and hence, an increase in anticoagulant effect. The fact that this scenario does not occur with sertraline, fluoxetine and paroxetine is compatible with an absence of effect of these 3 SSRIs on both CYP 1A2 and 2C9/10.

■ **CYP 2C9/10**

There have been no *in vitro* studies of the different effects of SSRIs on CYP 2C9/10. However, *in vivo* studies have been done with both tolbutamide and warfarin, which are substrates for this enzyme (Table 8.11). Fluoxetine and sertraline did not produce a clinically significant decrease in the clearance of tolbutamide or warfarin, and paroxetine did not affect warfarin.[16,159,245,273,287] Despite these results with fluoxetine, the U.S. Food and Drug Administration has compiled 163 cases in which the concomitant use of fluoxetine elevated phenytoin plasma levels. In 23 cases with adequate data, the average increase was 161%, occurring on average 2 weeks after fluoxetine was started, and was associated with development of clinical manifestations of toxicity including ataxia, somnolence and nystagmus.[71,134,249,293] These cases have led to a revision of the product labelling for fluoxetine to advise about this interaction. Since phenytoin is metabolized by CYP 2C9/10, this interaction suggests that fluoxetine inhibits this CYP enzyme. The reason for the apparent discrepancy between this effect of fluoxetine on phenytoin clearance and the absence of an effect of fluoxetine on the clearance of tolbutamide and warfarin is not known.

■ CYP 2C19

No *in vivo* studies have been done with SSRIs using an ideal model substrate for this CYP enzyme. However, studies with 3 SSRIs (ie, fluoxetine, fluvoxamine and sertraline) have been performed with diazepam which is principally dependent on CYP 2C19 for its metabolisms at least at low concentrations (Table 8.11). Demethylation of diazepam to desmethyldiazepam is the major route of elimination and is dependent on CYP 2C19 at the concentrations achieved on conventional low doses.[9,26,56,132,286] At higher concentrations, this demethylation can also be mediated by CYP 3A3/4.[10,294] Hydroxylation of diazepam to temazepam is typically a minor pathway and is mediated by CYP 3A3/4.[26,119]

Desmethyldiazepam undergoes C3-hydroxylation which may be mediated by a single, rate-limiting enzyme, CYP 2C19.[26,119] In contrast, C3-hydroxylation of diazepam is minimal at low drug concentrations, increases sigmoidally with increasing concentrations, and may be mediated entirely by CYP 3A3/4.[119]

Diazepam thus does not fulfill the criteria of a model substrate due to its multiple pathways mediated by more than one CYP enzyme. Nonetheless, the *in vivo* studies that have explored the potential interaction between these three SSRIs and diazepam does provide useful information on whether they inhibit either CYP 2C19 or 3A3/4. Since the metabolism of diazepam at low substrate concentrations appears to be principally mediated by CYP 2C19, and since the *in vivo* studies that follow were done with low doses of diazepam and hence, at low substrate concentrations, their findings suggest the delay in diazepam clearance produced by some SSRIs is due to an effect on CYP 2C19.

Fluvoxamine (average dose = 112 mg/day) produced on average a 280% and 41% increase in the area under curve (AUC) for diazepam and desmethyldiazepam respectively. The effect on diazepam represented a 65% reduction in its apparent clearance from 0.40 to 0.14 ml/min/kg and a marked prolongation in diazepam half-life from 51 to 118 hours ($p < 0.01$).[203] Fluoxetine, using a loading dose strategy (60 mg/d × 8 days) that would produce combined levels of fluoxetine and norfluoxetine approximately 20% to 30% lower than those that will occur at steady-state on 20 mg/day, produced a 40% increase in the AUC of diazepam.[160] Another study using only 30 mg/d × 7 days did not produce an increase in diazepam AUC.[159] This finding is consistent with the concentration-dependent nature of the effect since this loading dose strategy (30 mg/d × 7 days) would produce less than half the levels that would be expected under steady-state conditions on 20 mg/day. In contrast to fluvoxamine, fluoxetine (60 mg/d × 8 days) reduced the levels of metabolically derived desmethyldiazepam; which raises the possibility of a different MOA (ie, an effect on a different CYP enzyme such a CYP 3A3/4 rather than CYP 2C19). Further work is needed with fluoxetine and a more ideal substrate for CYP 2C19 to determine to what extent its effects on diazepam are due to an effect on CYP 2C19 versus CYP 3A3/4. Based on the study by Gardner and colleagues, sertraline under steady-state conditions on its usually effective, minimum dose of 50 mg/day will be expected to produce an appreciably smaller effect (ie, approximately 8% increase in AUC) than either fluvoxamine or fluoxetine.[99] Thus, these studies with these 3 SSRIs suggests that CYP 2C19 is inhibited potently by fluvoxamine, possibly weakly by fluoxetine, and trivially inhibited by sertraline at each drugs' usually effective, minimum, antidepressant dose. No comment can be made about the potential impact of citalopram or paroxetine on CYP 2C19 since appropriate studies have not been done.

■ CYP 2D6

A large number of drugs from different therapeutic classes are dependent on 2D6 for their metabolism including TCAs, codeine, several neuroleptics, β-blockers, and Type IC antiarrhythmics (Table 7.9). Of all the CYP enzymes, 2D6 has been studied most thoroughly with respect to the different effects of SSRIs on its functional activity (Table 8.7, Table 8.9 and Figure 8.2). Based on most *in vitro* studies (Table 8.7), paroxetine is 2- to 4-times more potent than fluoxetine, and 5 to 20 times more potent than sertraline. Fluvoxamine and citalopram are also substantially less potent than paroxetine and fluoxetine with respect to the *in vitro* inhibition of 2D6.

Recall that fluoxetine is marketed as the racemate (Section 2). The *in vitro* data shown in Table 8.7 for the inhibition of CYP 2D6 is for the racemate. The potency of the two enantiomers of fluoxetine and norfluoxetine is shown in Table 8.10. The relative potency of these enantiomers for other CYP enzymes has not been established.

All of SSRIs, with the apparent exception of fluvoxamine, have "active" metabolites relative to the inhibition of this enzyme *in vitro* with a potency similar to that of the parent compound (Table 8.7). However, only norfluoxetine reaches sufficient concentrations at each drug's usually effective, minimum concentration under routine clinical conditions to contribute in a clinically meaningful way to the inhibition of this enzyme. The contribution of norfluoxetine takes on special significance due to its extended half-life (ie, 1 to 2 weeks), which means that the risk of a drug-drug interaction mediated by this active metabolite persists for weeks after fluoxetine has been discontinued.

FIGURE 8.2 — DIFFERENTIAL *IN VIVO* EFFECTS OF FIVE DIFFERENT SSRIS ON CYP 2D6 FUNCTION

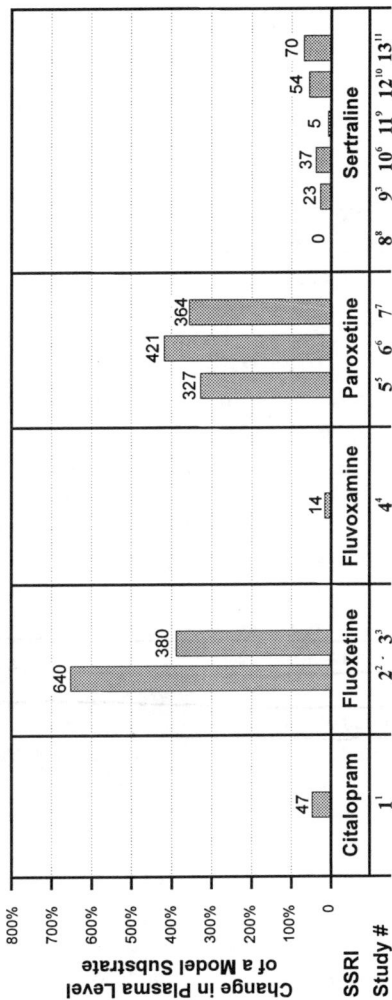

References: [1]110, [2]24, [3]219, [4]263, [5]4, [6]5, [7]41, [8]136, [9]264, [10]298, [11]153

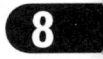

8

185

Desipramine has generally served as the model substrate for the *in vivo* studies of SSRIs on CYP 2D6 function (Table 8.9 and Figure 8.2). In these studies, the effect of each SSRI on the clearance of desipramine has been studied primarily at their usually effective dose: fluoxetine and paroxetine (20 mg/day) and sertraline (50 mg/day) (see Section 5). Since a fixed-dose study has not been published for citalopram or for fluvoxamine, their usually effective, minimum doses have not been as rigorously established (see Section 5). Nevertheless, they have been tested for effects on CYP 2D6 at doses of 40 mg/day for citalopram and 100 mg/day for fluvoxamine.

The results are quite clear about the relative impact of each SSRI on the *in vivo* clearance of desipramine: fluoxetine produced a 380% to 640% increase in desipramine levels; paroxetine, a 327% to 421% increase; citalopram, a 47% increase; sertraline, a 0% to 37% increase; and fluvoxamine, a 14% increase (Table 8.9, Figure 8.2). Thus, only 2 out of the 5 SSRIs marketed worldwide produce meaningful inhibition of this enzyme at their usually effective dose.

Only in the broadest sense can one state that all the SSRIs inhibit CYP 2D6. It is misleading to make such a claim without acknowledging the substantial differences among these drugs.

To further put the differences among the SSRIs in perspective, the above results for fluoxetine somewhat underestimate its full effect at steady-state at 20 mg/day. That is because steady-state levels of fluoxetine and norfluoxetine that would be expected at 20 mg/day were not achieved in either study due to the extended half-life of norfluoxetine. That is true even for the Bergstrom et al study which used a loading dose strategy of 60 mg/day for 7 days.

Only paroxetine and sertraline have been formally studied at doses above their usually effective dose. The study by Albers et al used a dose of 30 mg/day; however, that dose was administered for only 4 days prior to the administration of the test dose of imipramine.[4] Consistent with that short treatment phase, the plasma levels of paroxetine in this study (10-30 mg/ml) were similar to the 2 studies which gave 20 mg per day for at least 10 days.[5,41] Thus, the study by Albers et al was more of replication of those 2 earlier studies than a test of a higher dose.

Sertraline has been the one SSRI most extensively tested at doses above its usually effective antidepressant dose. Sproule et al found a 5% prolongation in the clearance of dextromethophan following treatment with sertraline 100 mg/day for 21 days.[264] Two separate studies examined the effect of sertraline 150 mg/day administered for a sufficient duration to achieve steady-state and found a 54% to 70% increase in desipramine plasma levels.[153,298] Thus sertraline at its usually effective dose of 50 mg/day produces a 0% to 37% increase in the plasma levels of a model substrate such as desipramine which is principally dependent on CYP 2D6 for its clearance, a 5% prolongation in clearance at 108 mg/day, and a 54% to 70% increase in plasma levels at 150 mg/day. The magnitude of this effect is substantially less at all of these doses than the effect of fluoxetine and paroxetine at their usually effective minimum dose.

While citalopram and fluvoxamine have been less extensively studied than sertraline, their effects on CYP 2D6 are also substantially less than fluoxetine and paroxetine (Table 8.9, Figure 8.2).

Figures 8.3 and 8.4 demonstrate the concentration-dependent nature of the effects of fluoxetine, paroxetine and sertraline on CYP 2D6 as reflected in the changes in plasma levels of the CYP 2D6 substrate, desipramine. These figures are from the formal *in vivo* pharmacokinetic studies that compared the effects of fluoxetine 20 mg/day to sertraline 50 mg/day in one study[219] and the effects of paroxetine 20 mg/day to

FIGURE 8.3 — TROUGH CONCENTRATIONS OF DESIPRAMINE IN PLASMA CORRELATED WITH CONCENTRATIONS OF SERTRALINE PLUS DESMETHYLSERTRALINE IN THE SERTRALINE TREATMENT GROUP AND FLUOXETINE PLUS NORFLUOXETINE IN THE FLUOXETINE TREATMENT GROUP

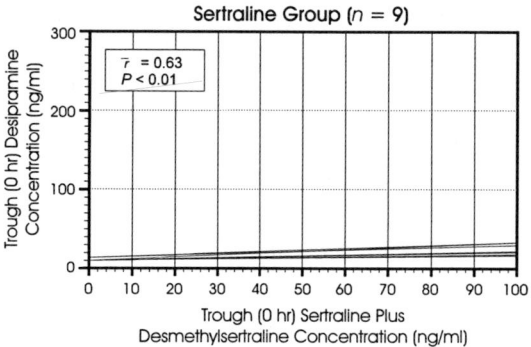

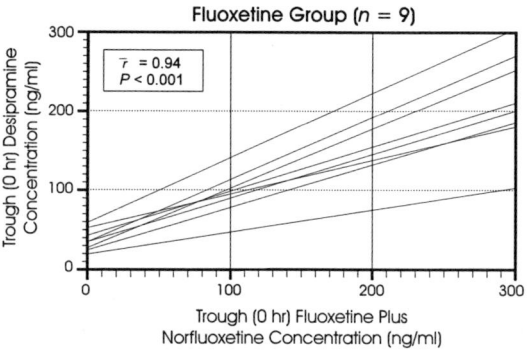

Sertraline Group ($n = 9$)

$\bar{r} = 0.63$
$P < 0.01$

Trough (0 hr) Desipramine Concentration (ng/ml)

Trough (0 hr) Sertraline Plus Desmethylsertraline Concentration (ng/ml)

Fluoxetine Group ($n = 9$)

$\bar{r} = 0.94$
$P < 0.001$

Trough (0 hr) Desipramine Concentration (ng/ml)

Trough (0 hr) Fluoxetine Plus Norfluoxetine Concentration (ng/ml)

Reference: 219

FIGURE 8.4 — TROUGH CONCENTRATIONS OF DESIPRAMINE IN PLASMA CORRELATED WITH CONCENTRATIONS OF SERTRALINE PLUS DESMETHYLSERTRALINE IN THE SERTRALINE TREATMENT GROUP AND PAROXETINE IN THE PAROXETINE TREATMENT GROUP

DMI = 967.5 × Sertraline + *N*-desmethylsertraline / (Sertraline + *N*-desmethylsertraline + 148.8)

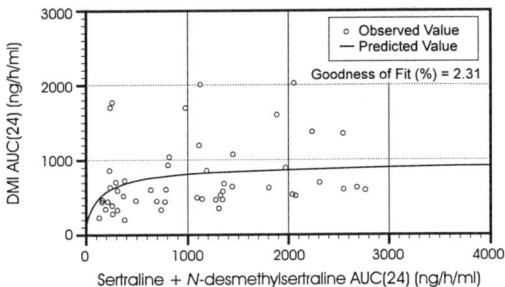

DMI = 6186.7 × Paroxetine / (Paroxetine + 677.7)

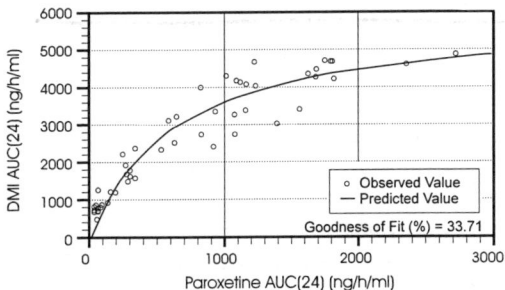

Michaelis-Menten Modeling of desipramine AUC(24) to sertraline + *N*-desmethylsertraline AUC(24) and Paroxetine AUC(24).

AUC = Area under curve.

Reference: 5

8

sertraline 50 mg/day in a second study.[5] On the X-axis of the graphs is the concentration of each respective SSRI and on the Y-axis is the plasma concentration of desipramine. There is a robust relationship between increasing plasma levels of fluoxetine plus norfluoxetine and increasing levels of desipramine in Figure 8.3. The same is true for paroxetine and desipramine plasma levels in Figure 8.4. In both figures, the relationship between increasing plasma levels of sertraline and elevations of desipramine plasma levels is considerably more modest. These results are fully consistent with the differences in the *in vitro* potency of these 3 SSRIs for the inhibition of CYP 2D6 and the differences in concentrations of 3 SSRIs at this enzyme at each drug's usually effective, minimum dose. Table 10.1 provides further illustration of the concentration-dependent nature of the inhibition of CYP enzymes.

To put these results in perspective, fluoxetine and paroxetine appear to produce approximately 85% inhibition of CYP 2D6 activity versus 15% inhibition or less with citalopram, fluvoxamine or sertraline (Table 8.4).

■ **CYP 3A3/4**

With the exception of citalopram, all of the SSRIs and their primary metabolites have been studied in terms of their *in vitro* effects on the metabolism of alprazolam, which is a substrate for the CYP 3A3/4 enzyme (Table 8.7). Fluvoxamine and norfluoxetine were the most potent *in vitro* inhibitors of the SSRIs. Sertraline and paroxetine were intermediate. Fluoxetine, the parent drug, was the weakest. To keep these results in perspective, the *in vitro* potency of both fluvoxamine and norfluoxetine are considerably less potent than the antifungal agent, ketoconazole.[278]

This antifungal agent can produce clinically serious elevations of terfenadine due to its inhibition of

CYP 3A3/4.[29,126,127,279,297] Based on the results of *in vitro* studies, coadministration of fluvoxamine and fluoxetine (due to norfluoxetine) would be predicted to cause more *in vivo* inhibition of CYP 3A3/4-dependent drug metabolism than would either paroxetine or sertraline due to the difference in plasma concentrations of these different agents at comparable antidepressant doses of each agent (Table 8.4 and Section 10, *Appendix*) but substantially less than ketoconazole.

Unfortunately, this prediction has only been partially tested by formal *in vivo* studies. The *in vivo* effects of fluoxetine and fluvoxamine on the clearance of alprazolam, a model substrate for CYP 3A3/4, has been tested *in vivo*, but similar studies have not been done with citalopram, paroxetine or sertraline (Table 8.11). Fluvoxamine (100 mg/day for 10 days) produced a doubling of alprazolam plasma levels with a 55% decrease in its clearance.[87] This finding is compatible with the *in vitro* data and the known plasma levels of fluvoxamine that would be expected at this dose.

In the first study with fluoxetine, a 33% increase in alprazolam plasma levels occurred after only 4 days of coadministration of fluoxetine 60 mg/day (ie, a loading dose strategy).[157] In the second study, the loading dose strategy for fluoxetine was 40 mg/day for 10 days which produced a combined plasma level of fluoxetine and norfluoxetine of 160 ng/ml, which is approximately 25% less than the steady-state levels of 200 ng/ml that should occur on 20 mg/day.[112] In this study, fluoxetine produced a 25% decrease in the clearance of alprazolam. Based on the results of these 2 studies, fluoxetine, at steady-state on 20 mg/day, will be expected to produce a 30% to 40% increase in alprazolam plasma levels. As with the inhibition of CYP 2D6, the effect of norfluoxetine on CYP 3A3/4 can last for an extended interval after fluoxetine discontinuation. In the second study, the increase in alprazolam plasma levels persisted for more than 2 weeks after nor-fluoxetine was discontinued.[112]

There have been some other studies relative to CYP 3A3/4 substrates which deserve some comment (Table 8.11). Carbamazepine is in part metabolized by CYP 3A3/4.[143,172,207] However, carbamazepine is not a model substrate due to the fact that it induces its own metabolism as well as the metabolism of other drugs. Thus, interaction studies with carbamazepine are not easily interpreted. With this caveat in mind, it is note-worthy that fluoxetine-induced slowing of carbamaz-epine metabolism has been reported by some but not all investigators.[101,102,113,201,261] There is also a case re-port describing cardiac abnormalities occurring 30 days after fluoxetine was added to a regimen containing terfenadine and resolved when terfenadine was stopped.[268] This case, coupled with the *in vitro* and *in vivo* data discussed above, suggests the need for a for-mal study given the widespread use of fluoxetine and terfenadine, coupled with the potential seriousness of a significant interaction. The available data suggest that fluoxetine at 20 mg/day is unlikely to produce sufficient inhibition of CYP 3A3/4 to produce a clini-cally significant interaction with terfenadine.

There are also case reports of 30% to 70% in-creases in carbamazepine levels when 100 to 300 mg/day of fluvoxamine is coadministered.[35,96] In a formal study, sertraline at a dose of 200 mg/day (which is four-times its usually effective, minimum dose) did not al-ter carbamazepine levels.[74] In a controlled-case series as opposed to a formal pharmacokinetic study, paroxetine did not alter carbamazepine levels.[8]

Taken as a whole, these studies indicate that CYP 3A3/4 inhibition produced by SSRIs at their usually effective dose ranges from moderate to not detectable as follows: fluvoxamine (moderate) > fluoxetine (mild) > paroxetine and sertraline (not detectable) (Table 8.7). There are a few caveats to this statement.

TABLE 8.11 — COMPARISON OF THE *IN VIVO* EFFECTS OF DIFFERENT SSRIS ON SPECIFIC CYP ENZYME SUBSTRATES*

| SSRI | Changes in Plasma Levels | | | | |
| | CYP 2C9/10 | | CYP 2C19 | CYP 3A3/4 | |
	TBA	PHT	DZ	APZ	CBZ
Fluoxetine	↑ 4%[1]	↑ 161%[2]	50%[3]	↑ 33%[4] ↑ 26%[5]	27%[6] 0-63%[7]
Fluvoxamine	NA	NA	↑ 300%[8]	↑ 100%[9]	30-70%[10]
Paroxetine	0%[11]	NA	NA	NA	0%[12]
Sertraline	≈ 5%[13]	0%[14]	≈ 3%[15]	NA	0%[16]

* CYP 2C9/10: TBA = tolbutamide, PHT = phenytoin
  CYP 2C19: DZ = diazepam
  CYP 3A3/4: APZ = alprazolam, CBZ = carbamazepine

[1] Formal *in vivo* study, 30 mg/d × 8 days, an inadequate loading dose strategy.[159]
[2] Large number of case reports with doses generally 20 mg/d for weeks.[71,134,249,293]
[3] Formal *in vivo* study, 60 mg/d × 8 days.[160]
[4] Formal *in vivo* study, 60 mg/d × 4 days.[157]
[5] Formal *in vivo* study, 40 mg/d × 7 days.[112]
[6] Formal *in vivo* study, 20 mg/d × 7 days.[113]
[7] Large number of case reports with doses generally approximately 20 mg/d at steady-state.[101,201,261]
[8] Formal *in vivo* study, 112 mg/d × 16 days.[203]
[9] Formal *in vivo* study, 100 m/d × 10 days.[87]
[10] Large number of case reports with doses of 100-300 mg/d.[35,96]
[11] Formal *in vivo* study, 30 mg/d × 10 days. While there was a non-significant increase in warfarin AUC, 5 out of 27 experienced increased bleeding.[16]
[12] Controlled-case series, 30 mg/d × 10 days.[8]
[13] Formal *in vivo* study, 200 mg/d × 16 days caused an 18% increase which would be approximately 5% at its usually effective dose of 50 mg/d.[273]
[14] Formal *in vivo* study, 200 mg/d × 16 days. No significant change.[65]
[15] Formal *in vivo* study, 200 mg/d × 16 days caused a 13% increase which would be approximately 3% at its usually effective dose of 50 mg/d.[99]
[16] Formal *in vivo* study, 200 mg/d × 16 days caused a nonsignificant decrease.[74]

8

First, citalopram is not mentioned because it has not been studied adequately. Second, the effects on these enzymes is concentration dependent so that higher doses could produce greater effect. This is particularly important for SSRIs, which have nonlinear pharmacokinetics (see Section 7). For example, fluoxetine produces mild inhibition of CYP 3A3/4 at 20 mg/day, but will be expected to increase disproportionately with dose increases. The mild inhibition (20% to 50% change) will not be expected to produce a clinically meaningful drug-drug interaction in most instances, but the likelihood and severity of a clinically meaningful interaction increases as the magnitude of the change in clearance due to the degree of enzyme inhibition increases (see Appendix).

To put these results in perspective, it is important to recognize the substantial difference between the inhibition produced by fluvoxamine and fluoxetine and the effects of drugs such as ketoconazole. That has unfortunately not been done in several recent review articles.[301,302] These papers have listed several SSRIs as inhibitors of CYP 3A3/4 along with drugs such as ketoconazole without acknowledging the difference in the magnitude of their effects. The profound inhibition of CYP 3A3/4 enzyme produced by ketoconazole and itraconazole is responsible for the potentially fatal interaction of these drugs with terfenadine. While fluvoxamine is the most potent SSRI *in vitro* with regard to CYP 3A3/4 inhibition, it is three orders of magnitude less potent than ketoconazole. *In vivo* studies have confirmed that there is a 20- to 100-fold difference between the effects of fluvoxamine and fluoxetine on the CYP 3A3/4 mediated biotransformation of model substrates such as triazolobenzodiazepines and the effects of antifungal agents such as ketoconazole and itraconazole under clinically relevant dosing conditions (Figure 8.5). Failure to recognize these substantial differences can cause significant confusion about the relative risk of experiencing a serious adverse drug-drug interaction due to CYP 3A3/4 inhibition.

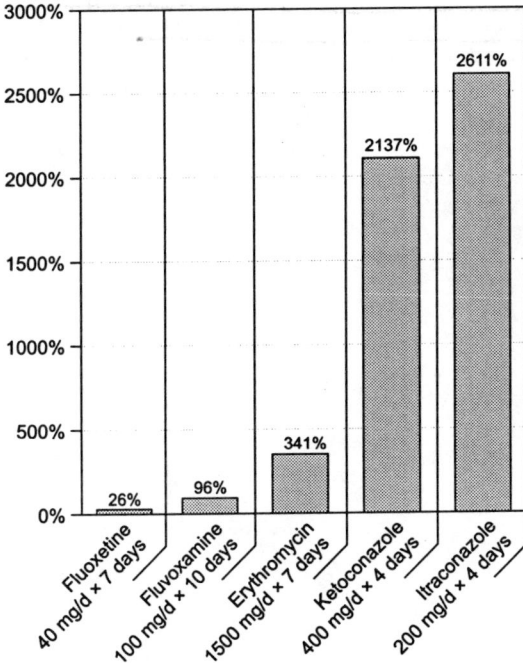

FIGURE 8.5 — RELATIVE *IN VIVO* EFFECTS OF CYP 3A3/4 INHIBITORS ON TRIAZOLOBENZODIAZEPINES (TBZ)

Percent Increase in Plasma Drug Levels of TBZs (AUC)

	Percent Increase
Fluoxetine 40 mg/d × 7 days	26%
Fluvoxamine 100 mg/d × 10 days	96%
Erythromycin 1500 mg/d × 7 days	341%
Ketoconazole 400 mg/d × 4 days	2137%
Itraconazole 200 mg/d × 4 days	2611%

AUC = Area under curve.

References: 303-306

8

195

Table 8.11 summarizes the *in vivo* data which is available for the 4 most extensively studied SSRIs in terms of their effects on CYP enzymes other than CYP 2D6. The results for CYP 2D6 are summarized in Table 8.9 and Figure 8.2. Since the inhibition of these enzymes is concentration-dependent, it is important to ensure an adequate trial of the usually effective, minimum dose, particularly for SSRIs such as fluvoxamine and fluoxetine which inhibit more than one CYP enzyme. The data are clear that the effect of the SSRIs on specific CYP enzymes is an SSRI-specific issue rather than a class issue and involves considerations beyond the *in vitro* inhibition constant (K_i) as further discussed in Section 10, *Appendix*.

9 References

1. Aberg-Wistedt A. Comparison between zimelidine and desipramine in endogenous depression: a cross-over study. *Acta Psychiatr Scan*. 1982;66:129-138.

2. Aberg-Wistedt A. The antidepressant effects of 5-HT uptake inhibitors. *Br J Psychiatry*. 1989;155(suppl 8):32-40.

3. Agundez JAG, Martinez C, Ladero JM, et al. Pharmacokinetics and drug disposition: debrisoquine oxidation genotype and susceptibility to lung cancer. *Clin Pharmacol Ther*. 1994;55:10-14.

4. Albers LJ, Reist C, Helmeste D, Vu R, Jang SW. Paroxetine shifts imipramine metabolism. *Psychiatry Research*. 1996; 59:189-196.

5. Alderman J, Greenblatt D, Allison J, Preskorn S, Harrison W, Chung M. Desipramine pharmacokinetics with the selective serotonin reuptake inhibitors (SSRIs), paroxetine or sertraline. Poster presented at the American Psychiatric Association Sesquicentennial Celebration, 1844-1994; May 21-26, 1994; Philadelphia, Pa.

6. Altamura AC, Montgomery SA, Wernicke JF. The evidence for 20 mg a day of fluoxetine as the optimal dose in the treatment of depression. *Br J Psychiatry*. 1988;153 (suppl 3):109-112.

7. Altamura AC, Moro AR, Percudani M. Clinical pharmacokinetics of fluoxetine. *Clin Pharmacokinet*. 1994;26: 201-214.

8. Andersen BB, Mikkelsen M, Vesterager A, et al. No influence of the antidepressant paroxetine on carbamazepine valproate and phenytoin. *Epilepsy Res*. 1991:201-204.

9. Andersson T. Omeprazole drug interaction studies. *Clin Pharmacokinet*. 1991;21:195-212.

10.   Andersson T, Miners JO, Veronese ME, Birkett DJ. Diaz-
        epam metabolism by human liver microsomes is mediated
        by both *S*-mephenytoin hydroxylase and CYP3A isoforms.
        Br J Clin Pharmacol. 1994;38:131-137.

11.   Aronoff GR, Bergstrom RF, Pottratz ST, Sloan RS, Wolen
        RL, Lemberger L. Fluoxetine kinetics and protein binding
        in normal and impaired renal function. *Clin Pharmacol
        Ther.* 1984;36:138-144.

12.   Baker GB, Coutts RT, Holt A. Metabolism and chirality in
        psychopharmacology. *Biol Psychiatry.* 1994;36:211-213.
        Editorial.

13.   Balant LP. Pharmacokinetics in special populations. Pre-
        sented at *European Psychopharmacology Consensus Meet-
        ing* as a satellite meeting to the First International Congress
        on Hormones, Brain and Neuropsychopharmacology; Sep-
        tember 13-17, 1993; Rhodes, Greece.

14.   Balant-Gorgia AE, Balant LP, Genet C, Dayer P, Aeschli-
        mann JM, Garrone G. Importance of oxidative poly-
        morphism and levomepromazine treatment on the steady-
        state blood concentrations of clomipramine and its major
        metabolites. *Eur J Clin Pharmacol.* 1986;31:449-455.

15.   Balant-Gorgia AE, Schulz P, Dayer P, et al. Role of oxida-
        tion polymorphism on blood and urine concentrations of
        amitriptyline and its metabolites in man. *Arch Psychiatr
        Nervenki.* 1982;232:215-222.

16.   Bannister SJ, Houser VP, Hulse JD, Kisicki JC, Rasmussen
        JGC. Evaluation of the potential for interactions of
        paroxetine with diazepam, cimetidine, warfarin, and
        digoxin. *Acta Psychiatr Scand.* 1989;80(suppl 350):102-
        106.

17.   Barbeau A, Roy M, Paris S, Cloutier T, Plasse L, Poirier J.
        Ecogenetics of Parkinson's disease: 4-hydroxylation of
        debrisoquine. *Lancet.* 1985;2:1213-1216.

18.   Baumann P, Bertschy G. Pharmacodynamic and pharmaco-
        kinetic interactions of selective serotonin reuptake inhib-
        iting antidepressants (SSRIs) with other psychotropic
        drugs. *Nord J Psychiatry.* 1993;47(suppl 30):13-19.

19. Baumann P, Jonzier-Perey M, Koeb L, Kupfer A, Tinguely D, Schopf J. Amitriptyline pharmacokinetics and clinical response: II. Metabolic polymorphism assessed by hydroxylation of debrisoquine and mephenytoin. *Intl Clin Psychopharmacol.* 1986;1:102-112.

20. Baumann P, Rochat B. Comparative pharmacokinetics of selective serotonin reuptake inhibitors: a look behind the mirror. *Intl Clin Psychopharmacol.* 1995;10(suppl 1):15-21.

21. Bayer AJ, Roberts NA, Allen EA, et al. The pharmacokinetics of paroxetine in the elderly. *Acta Psychiatr Scan.* 1989;80(suppl 350):85-86.

22. Benfield P, Ward A. Fluvoxamine: a review of its pharmacodyamic and pharmacokinetic properties, and therapeutic efficacy in depressive illness. *Drugs.* 1986; 32:313-334.

23. Bergstrom RF, Lemberger L, Farid NA, Wolen RL. Clinical pharmacology and pharmacokinetics of fluoxetine: a review. *Br J Psychiatry.* 1988;153(suppl 3):47-50.

24. Bergstrom RF, Peyton AL, Lemberger L. Quantification and mechanism of the fluoxetine and tricyclic antidepressant interaction. *Clin Pharmacol Ther.* 1992;51:239-248.

25. Bertilsson L, Aberg-Wistedt A. The debrisoquine hydroxylation test predicts steady-state plasma levels of desipramine. *Br J Clin Pharmacol.* 1983;15:388-390.

26. Bertilsson L, Henthorn TK, Sanz E, Tybring G, Sawe J, Villen T. Importance of genetic factors in the regulation of diazepam metabolism: relationship to *S*-mephenytoin, but not debrisoquine, hydroxylation phenotype. *Clin Pharmacol Ther.* 1989;45:348-355.

27. Bertschy G, Vandel S, Allers G, Volmat R. Fluvoxamine-tricyclic antidepressant interaction. *Eur J Clin Pharmacol.* 1991;40:119-120.

28. Bertschy G, Vandel S, Francois T, et al. Metabolic interaction between tricyclic antidepressant and fluvoxamine and fluoxetine, a pharmacogenetic approach. *Clin Neuropharm.* 1992;15(suppl 1):78A-79A.

9

29.   Biglin KE, Faraon MS, Constance TD, Lieh-Lai M. Drug-induced torsades de pointes: a possible interaction of terfenadine and erythromycin. *Ann Pharmacother*. 1994; 28:282.

30.   Birgersson C, Morgan ET, Jornvall H, von Bahr C. Purification of a desmethylimipramine and debrisoquine hydroxylating cytochrome P450 from human liver. *Biochem Pharmacol*. 1986;35:3165-3166.

31.   Bjerkenstedt L, Flyckt L, Overo KF, Lingjaerde O. Relationship between clinical effects, serum drug concentration and serotonin uptake inhibition in depressed patients treated with citalopram. A double-blind comparison of three dose levels. *Eur J Clin Pharmacol*. 1985;28:553-557.

32.   Bloomer JC, Woods FR, Haddock RE, Lennard MS, Tucker GT. The role of cytochrome P4502D6 in the metabolism of paroxetine by human liver microsomes. *Br J Clin Pharmacol*. 1992;33:521-523.

33.   Boehnert MT, Lovejoy FH. Value of the QRS duration versus serum drug level in predicting seizures and ventricular arrhythmias after an acute overdose of tricyclic antidepressants. *N Engl J Med*. 1985;313:474-479.

34.   Bolden-Watson C, Richelson E. Blockade by newly-developed antidepressants of biogenic amine uptake into rat brain synaptosomes. *Life Sci*. 1993;52:1023-1029.

35.   Bonnet P, Vandel S, Nezelog S, Sechter D, Bizouard P. Carbamazepine, fluvoxamine: is there a pharmacokinetic interaction? *Therapie*. 1992;47:165.

36.   Borys DJ, Setzer SC, Ling LJ, et al. Acute fluoxetine overdose: a report of 234 cases. *Am J Emerg Med*. 1992;10: 115-120.

37.   Bouquet S, Vandel S, Bertschy G, et al. Pharmacokinetics of fluoxetine and fluvoxamine in depressed patients: personal results. *Clin Neuropharmacol*. 1992;15(suppl 1): 82A-83A.

38.   Breyer-Pfaff U, Pfandl B, Nill K, et al. Enantioselective amitriptyline metabolism in patients phenotyped for two cytochrome P450 isoenzymes. *Clin Pharmacol Ther*. 1992; 52:350-358.

39. Brøsen K. Isozyme specific drug oxidation: genetic polymorphism and drug-drug interactions. *Nord J Psychiatry*. 1993;47(suppl 30):21-26.

40. Brøsen K. Recent developments in hepatic drug oxidation: implications for clinical pharmacokinetics. *Clin Pharmacokinet*. 1990;18:220-239.

41. Brøsen K, Hansen JG, Nielsen KK, Sindrup SH, Gram LF. Inhibition by paroxetine of desipramine metabolism in extensive but not in poor metabolizers of sparteine. *Eur J Clin Pharmacol*. 1993;44:349-355.

42. Brøsen K, Gram LF. Quinidine inhibits the 2-hydroxylation of imipramine and desipramine but not the demethylation of imipramine. *Eur J Clin Pharmacol*. 1989;37:155-160.

43. Brøsen K, Gram LF, Kragh-Sorensen P. Extremely slow metabolism of amitriptyline but normal metabolism of imipramine and desipramine in an extensive metabolizer of sparteine, debrisoquine, and mephenytoin. *Ther Drug Monit*. 1991;13:177-182.

44. Brøsen K, Gram LF, Sindrup S, Skjelbo E, Nielson KK. Pharmacogenetics of tricyclic and novel antidepressants: recent developments. *Clin Neuropharm*. 1992;15(suppl 1): 80A-81A.

45. Brøsen K, Klysner R, Gram LF, Otton SV, Bech P, Bertilsson L. Steady-state concentrations of imipramine and its metabolites in relation to the sparteine/debrisoquine polymorphism. *Eur J Clin Pharmacol*. 1986;30:679-684.

46. Brøsen K, Otton SV, Gram LF. Imipramine demethylation and hydroxylation: impact of the sparteine oxidation phenotype. *Clin Pharmacol Ther*. 1986;40:543-549.

47. Brøsen K, Skjelbo E, Rasmussen BB, Puolsen HE, Loft S. Fluvoxamine is a potent inhibitor of cytochrome P4501A2. *Biochem Pharmacol*. 1993;45:1211-1214.

48. Brøsen K, Zeugin T, Meyer UA. Role of P4502D6, the target of the sparteine-debrisoquine oxidation polymorphism, in the metabolism of imipramine. *Clin Pharmacol Ther*. 1991;49:609-617.

9

49.   Burke MJ, Silkey B, Preskorn SH. Pharmacoeconomic considerations when evaluating treatment options for major depressive disorder. *J Clin Psychiatry*. 1994;55 (suppl A): 42-52.

50.   Butler M, Lang N, Young J, et al. Determination of CYP 1A2 and NAT2 phenotypes in human populations by analysis of caffeine urinary metabolites. *Pharmacogenetics*. 1992;2:116-127.

51.   Cade JFJ. Lithium salts in the treatment of psychotic excitement. *Med J Aust*. 1949;2:349-352.

52.   Callaham M, Kassel D. Epidemiology of fatal tricyclic antidepressant ingestion: implications for management. *Ann Emer Med*. 1985;14:1-9.

53.   Caporaso N, Hayes RB, Dosemeci M, et al. Lung cancer risk, occupational exposure, and the debrisoquine metabolic phenotype. *Cancer Res*. 1989;49:3675-3679.

54.   Caporaso N, Landi MT, Vineis P. Relevance of metabolic polymorphisms to human carcinogenesis: evaluation of epidemiologic evidence. *Pharmacogenetics*. 1991;1:4-19.

55.   Caporaso NE, Tucker MA, Hoover RN, et al. Lung cancer and the debrisoquine metabolic phenotype. *J Natl Cancer Inst*. 1990;82:1264-1272.

56.   Caraco Y, Tateishi T, Wood AJJ. Ethnic effects on inhibition of drug metabolism. *Clin Pharmacol Ther*. 1994;55: 169. Abstract.

57.   Cardiac Arrhythmia Pilot Study (CAPS) Investigators. Effects of encainide, flecainide, imipramine and moricizine on ventricular arrhythmias during the year after acute myocardial infarction: the CAPS. *Am J Cardiol*. 1988;61: 501-509.

58.   Chiba K, Saitoh A, Koyama E, Tani M, Hayashi M, Ishizaki T. The role of *S*-mephenytoin 4'-hydroxylase in imipramine metabolism by human liver microsomes: a two-enzyme kinetic analysis of *N*-demethylation and 2-hydroxylation. *Br J Clin Pharmacol*. 1994;37:237-242.

59. Clomipramine hydrochloride (Anafranil). *Physicians' Desk Reference.* 49th ed. Montvale, NJ: Medical Economics Data Production Company; 1995:596-599.

60. Clozapine (Clozaril). *Physicians' Desk Reference.* 49th ed. Montvale, NJ: Medical Economics Data Production Company; 1995:2149-2153.

61. Cooper RG, Evans DAP, Whibley EJ. Polymorphic hydroxylation of perhexiline maleate in man. *J Med Genet.* 1984;21:27-33.

62. Coulehan JL, Schulberg HC, Block MR, et al. Depressive symptomatology and medical co-morbidity in a primary care clinic. *Intl J Psychiatry Med.* 1990;20:335-347.

63. Crane GE. Iproniazid (Marsilid) phosphate, a therapeutic agent for mental disorders and debilitating disease. *Psychiatry Res Rep.* 1957;8:142-152.

64. Crewe HK, Lennard MS, Tucker GT, Woods FR, Haddock RE. The effect of paroxetine and other specific serotonin reuptake inhibitors on cytochrome P450IID6 activity in human liver microsomes. *Br J Clin Pharmacol.* 1991;32:658P-659P.

65. Rapeport WG, Muirhead DC, Williams SA, Cross M, Wesnes K. Absence of effect of sertraline on the pharmacokinetics and pharmacodynamics of phenytoin. *J Clin Psychiatry.* 1996;57(suppl 1):24-28.

66. Cusack B, Nelson A, Richelson E. Binding of antidepressants to human brain receptors: focus on newer generation compounds. *Psychopharmacol.* 1994;114:559-565.

67. Dahl M, Nordin C, Bertilsson L. Enantioelective hydroxylation of nortriptyline in human liver microsomes, intestinal homogenate, and patients treated with nortriptyline. *Ther Drug Monit.* 1991;13:189-194.

68. Dalhoff K, Almdal TP, Bjerrum K, et al. Paroxetine in patients with cirrhosis. *Psychopharmacol.* 1991;103:B13.

69. Danish University Antidepressant Group. Citalopram: clinical effect profile in comparison with clomipramine: a controlled multicenter study. *Psychopharmacol.* 1986; 90:131-138.

70. Danish University Antidepressant Group. Paroxetine: a selective serotonin reuptake inhibitor showing better tolerance, but weaker antidepressant effect than clomipramine in a controlled multicenter study. *J Affective Disorder*. 1990;18:289-299.

71. Darley J. Interaction between phenytoin and fluoxetine. *Seizure*. 1994;3:151-152.

72. Davidson J. Seizures and bupropion: a review. *J Clin Psychiatry*. 1989;50:256-261.

73. de Vries MH, Raghoebar M, Mathlener IS, van Harten J. Single and multiple oral dose fluvoxamine kinetics in young and elderly subjects. *Ther Drug Monit*. 1992;14: 493-498.

74. Rapeport WG, Williams SA, Muirhead DC, Dewland PM, Tanner T, Wesnes K. Absence of a sertraline-mediated effect on the pharmacokinetics and pharmacodynamics of carbamazepine. *J Clin Psychiatry*. 1996;57(suppl 1):20-23.

75. Doogan DP, Caillard V. Sertraline in the prevention of depression. *Br J Psychiatry*. 1992;160:217-222.

76. Dorian P, Sellers EM, Reed KL, et al. Amitriptyline and ethanol: pharmacokinetic and pharmacodynamic interaction. *Eur J Clin Pharmacol*. 1983;25:325-331.

77. Dornseif BE, Dunlop SR, Potvin JH, Wernicke JF. Effect of dose escalation after low-dose fluoxetine therapy. *Psychopharmacol Bull*. 1989;25:71-79.

78. Doyle GD, Laher M, Kelly JG, et al. The pharmacokinetics of paroxetine in renal impairment. *Acta Psychiatr Scand*. 1989;80(suppl 350):89-90.

79. Dufour H, Bouchacourt M, Thermoz P, et al. Citalopram—a highly selective 5-HT reuptake inhibitor—in the treatment of depressed patients. *Intl Clin Psychopharmacol*. 1987;2:225-237.

80. Dunner DL, Dunbar GC. Optimal dose regimen for paroxetine. *J Clin Psychiatry*. 1992;53(suppl 2):21-26.

81. Emrich HM, Berger M, Riemann D, von Zerssen D. Serotonin reuptake inhibition versus norepinephrine reuptake

inhibition: a double-blind differential therapeutic study with fluvoxamine and oxaprotiline in endogenous and neurotic depressives. *Pharmacopsychiatrica.* 1987;20:60-63.

82. Eric LT. A prospective double-blind comparative multicentre study of paroxetine and placebo in preventing recurrent major depression episodes. *Biol Psychiatry.* 1991; 29(suppl 11):2545.

83. Evans D. Antidepressant adverse effects and antidepressants in the medically ill. *Am Soc Clin Psychopharm Progress Notes.* 1995;6:22-25.

84. Evans DA, Mahgoub A, Sloan TP, Idle JR, Smith RL. A family and population study of the genetic polymorphism of debrisoquine oxidation in a white British population. *J Med Genet.* 1980;17:102-105.

85. Fabre LF, Abuzzahab FS, Amin M, et al. Sertraline safety and efficacy in major depression: a double-blind fixed-dose comparison with placebo. *Biol Psychiatry.* 1995;38:592-602.

86. Feighner JP, Cohn JB. Double-blind comparative trials of fluoxetine and doxepin in geriatric patients with major depressive disorder. *J Clin Psychiatry.* 1985;46:20-25.

87. Fleishaker JC, Hulst LK. A pharmacokinetic and pharmacodynamic evaluation of the combined administration of alprazolam and fluvoxamine. *Eur J Clin Pharmacol.* 1994; 46:35-39.

88. Fleming CM, Kaisary A, Wilkinson GR, Smith P, Branch RA. The ability to 4-hydroxylate debrisoquine is related to recurrence of bladder cancer. *Pharmacogenetics.* 1992; 2:128-134.

89. Fluvoxamine maleate (Luvox). *Compendium of Pharmaceuticals and Specialities.* 30th ed. Ottawa, Ontario, Canada: Canadian Pharmaceutical Association; 1995:737-738.

90. Folgia JP, Perel JM, Nathan RS, Pollock BG. Therapeutic drug monitoring (TDM) of fluvoxamine, a selective antidepressant. *Clin Chem.* 1990;36:1043. Abstract.

9

91. Fonne-Pfister R, Bargetzi MJ, Meyer UA. MPTP, the neurotoxin inducing Parkinson's disease, is a potent competitive inhibitor of human and rat cytochrome P450 isozymes (P450 buf-I, P450 dbl) catalyzing debrisoquine 4-hydroxylation. *Biochem Biophys Res Comm.* 1987;148: 1144-1150.

92. Frank E, Kupfer DJ, Perel JM, et al. Three year outcomes for maintenance therapies in recurrent depression. *Arch Gen Psych.* 1990;47:1093-1099.

93. Fredricson OK. Kinetics of citalopram in man: plasma levels in patients. *Prog NeuroPsychopharmacol Biol Psychiatry.* 1982;6:311-318.

94. Fredericson OK. Preliminary studies of the kinetics of citalopram in man. *Eur J Clin Pharm.* 1978;14:69-73.

95. Fredericson OK, Toft B, Christophersen L, Gylding-Sabroe JP. Kinetics of citalopram in elderly patients. *Psychopharmacol.* 1985;86:253-257.

96. Fritze J, Unsorg B, Lanczik M. Interaction between carbamazepine and fluvoxamine. *Acta Psychiatr Scand.* 1991;84:583-584.

97. Frommer DA, Kulig DA, Marx JA, Rumack B. Tricyclic antidepressant overdose: a review. *JAMA.* 1987;257:521-526.

98. Fuller RW, Snoddy HD, Krushinski JH, Robertson DW. Comparison of norfluoxetine enantiomers as serotonin uptake inhibitors *in vivo. Neuropsychopharmacol.* 1992; 31:997-1000.

99. Gardner MJ, Ronfeld RA, Wilner KD, et al. Absence of a clinically meaningful effect of sertraline on the pharmacokinetics and protein binding of diazepam in healthy volunteers. *Clin Pharmacokinet.* In press.

100. Garnier R, Azoyan P, Chataigner D, Taboulet P, Dellattre D, Efthymiou ML. Acute fluvoxamine poisoning. *J Intern Med Res.* 1993;21:197-208.

101. Gernaat HBPE, Van De Woude J, Touw DJ. Fluoxetine and parkinsonism in patients taking carbamazepine. *Am J Psychiatry.* 1991;148:1604-1605.

102. Gidal BE, Anderson GD, Seaton TL, Miyoshi HR, Wilenksy AJ. Evaluation of the effect of fluoxetine on the formation of carbamazepine epoxide. *Ther Drug Monit.* 1993;15:405-409.

103. Glassman AH, Roose SP, Giardina EGV, Bigger JT Jr. Cardiovascular effects of tricyclic antidepressants. In: Meltzer HY, ed. *Psychopharmacology: The Third Generation of Progress.* New York, NY: Raven Press; 1987: 1437-1442.

104. Goldstein JA, de Morais SM. Biochemistry and molecular biology of the human CYP 2C subfamily. *Pharmacogenetics.* 1994;4:285-299.

105. Gonzalez FJ. Human cytochromes P450: problems and prospects. *Trends Pharmacol Sci.* 1992;13:346-352.

106. Gonzalez FJ, Gelboin HV. Human cytochromes P450: evolution and cDNA-directed expression. *Environmental Health Perspectives.* 1992;98:81-85.

107. Gonzalez FJ, Nebert DW. Evolution of the P450 gene superfamily: animal-plans "warfare," molecular drive and human genetic differences in drug oxidation. *Trends Genetics.* 1990;6:182-186.

108. Goodnick PJ. Pharmacokinetics of second generation of antidepressants: fluoxetine. *Psychopharm Bull.* 1991;27: 503-512.

109. Gram L, Brøsen K, Kragh-Sorensen P, Christensen P. Steady-state plasma levels of E- and Z-10-OH-nortriptyline in nortriptyline-treated patients: significance of concurrent mediation and the sparteine oxidation phenotype. *Ther Drug Monit.* 1989;11:508-514.

110. Gram LF, Hansen MGJ, Sindrup SH, et al. Citalopram: interaction studies with levomepromazine, imipramine, and lithium. *Ther Drug Monit.* 1993;15:18-24.

111. Greb WH, Buscher G, Dierdorf HD, Koster FE, Wolf D, Mellows G. The effect of liver enzyme inhibition by cimetidine and enzyme induction by phenobarbitone on the pharmacokinetics of paroxetine. *Acta Psychiatr Scand.* 1989;80(suppl 350):95-98.

9

112. Greenblatt DJ, Preskorn SH, Cotreau MM, Horst WD, Harmatz JS. Fluoxetine impairs clearance of alprazolam but not of clonazepam. *Clin Pharmacol Ther*. 1992;52:479-486.

113. Grimsley SR, Jann MW, Carter JG, D'Mello AP, D'Souza MJ. Increased carbamazepine plasma concentrations after fluoxetine coadministration. *Clin Pharmacol Ther*. 1991; 50:10-15.

114. Guengerich FP. Bioactivation and detoxication of toxic and carginogenic chemicals. *Drug Metab Dispos*. 1993; 21:1-6.

115. Guengerich FP. Cytochrome P450 enzymes. *Am Scientist*. 1993;81:440-447.

116. Guengerich FP. Human cytochrome P450 enzymes. *Life Sci*. 1992;50:1471-1478.

117. Guengerich FP, Shimada T. Oxidation of toxic and carcinogenic chemicals by human cytochrome P450 enzymes. *Chem Res Toxicol*. 1991;4:391-407.

118. Hartter S, Wetzel H, Hammes E, Hiemke C. Inhibition of antidepressant demethylation and hydroxylation by fluvoxamine in depressed patients. *Psychopharmacol*. 1993; 110:302-308.

119. Harvey A, Preskorn S. Cytochrome P450 enzymes: interpretation of their interactions with SSRIs. *J Clin Psychopharm*. In press.

120. Harvey AT, Preskorn SH. Interactions of serotonin reuptake inhibitors with tricyclic antidepressants. *Arch Gen Psychiatry*. 1995;52:783-784.

121. Hayashi S, Watanabe J, Nakachi K, Kawajiri K. Genetic linkage of lung cancer-associated MspI polymorphisms with amino acid replacement in the hemo binding region of the human cytochrome P4501A1 gene. *J Biochem*. 1991; 110:407-411.

122. Hebenstreit GF, Fellerer K, Zochling R, Zentz A, Dunbar GC. A pharmacokinetic dose titration study in adult and elderly depressed patients. *Acta Psychiatr Scand*. 1989;80 (suppl 350):81-84.

123. Hindmarch I, Subhan Z, Stoker MJ. The effects of zimelidine and amitriptyline on car driving and psychomotor performance. *Acta Psychiatr Scand*. 1983;68(suppl 308):141-146.

124. Hiramatsu KT, Takahashi R, Mori A, et al. A multicentre, double-blind comparative trial of zimelidine and imipramine in primary major depressive disorders. *Acta Psychiatr Scand*. 1983;68(suppl 308):41-54.

125. Holm M, Olesen F. Psykofarmakordination i almen praksis (Prescribing of psychotropic drugs in general practice). *Ugskr Laeger*. 1989;151:2122-2126.

126. Honig PK, Woosley RL, Zamani K, Conner DP, Cantilena LR Jr. Changes in the pharmacokinetics and eletrocardiographic pharmacodynamics of terfenadine with concomitant administration of erythromycin. *Clin Pharmacol Ther*. 1992;52:231-238.

127. Honig PK, Wortham DC, Zamani K, Conner DP, Mullin JC, Cantilena LR. Terfenadine-ketoconazole interaction. Pharmacokinetic and electrocardiographic consequences. *JAMA*. 1993;269:1513-1518.

128. Hoyer D, Clark DE, Fozard JR, et al. International Union of Pharmacology classification of receptors for 5-hydroxytryptamine (serotonin). *Pharmacol Rev*. 1994;46:157-203.

129. Hyttel J. Comparative pharmacology of selective serotonin reuptake inhibitors (SSRIs). *Nord J Psychiatry*. 1993;47 (suppl 30):5-12.

130. Hyttel J, Bogeso KP, Perregaard J, Sanchez C. The pharmacological effect of citalopram residues in the (S)-(+)-enantiomer. *J Neural Transm*. 1992;88:157-160.

131. Inaba T, Jurima M, Mahon WA, Kalow W. *In vitro* inhibition studies of two isozymes of human liver cytochrome P450: mephenytoin *P*-hydroxylase and sparteine monooxygenase. *Drug Metab Dispos*.1985;13:443-448.

132. Ishizaki T, Chiba K, Manabe K, et al. Comparison of the effects of E3810 and omeprazole on diazepam pharmacokinetics in extensive and poor metabolizers of *S*-mephenytoin. *Clin Pharmacol Ther*. 1994;55:141. Abstract.

133.   Jacobsen FM. SSRI-induced sexual dysfunction. *American Society of Clinical Psychopharmacology Progress Notes*. 1994;5:1-4.

134.   Jalil P. Toxic reaction following the combined administration of fluoxetine and phenytoin: two case reports. *J Neurol Neurosurg Psychiatry*. 1992;55:412-413.

135.   Janicak PG, Davis JM, Preskorn SH, Syd FJ Jr. *Principles and Practices of Psychopharmacotherapy*. Baltimore, Md: Williams and Wilkins; 1993.

136.   Jann MW, Carson SW, Grimsley SR, Erikson SM, Kumar A, Carter JG. Lack of effect of sertraline on the pharmacokinetics and pharmacodynamics of imipramine and its metabolites. *Clin Pharm Therap*. 1995;57:207. Abstract.

137.   Jerling M, Lindstrom L, Bondesson U, Bertilsson L. Fluvoxamine inhibition and carbamazepine induction of the metabolism of clozapine: evidence from a therapeutic drug monitoring service. *Ther Drug Monit*. 1994;16:368-374.

138.   Kaisary A, Smith P, Jaczq E, et al. Genetic predisposition to bladder cancer: ability to hydroxylate debrisoquine and mephenytoin as risk factors. *Cancer Res*. 1987;47:5488-5493.

139.   Kalow W, Tyndale RF. Debrisoquine/sparteine monooxygenase and other P450s in brain. In: Kalow W, ed. *Pharmacogenetics of Drug Metabolism*. New York, NY: Pergammon Press, Inc; 1992:649-656.

140.   Kasper S, Dotsch M, Vieira A, Kick H, Moller HJ. Plasma concentration of fluvoxamine and maprotiline in major depression: implications on therapeutic efficacy and side effects. *Eur Neuropsychopharm*. 1993;3:13-21.

141.   Kaye CM, Haddock RE, Langley PF, et al. A review of the metabolism and pharmacokinetics of paroxetine in man. *Acta Psychiatr Scand*. 1989;80(supp 350):60-75.

142.   Kelly MW, Perry PJ, Holstad SG, Garvey MJ. Serum fluoxetine and norfluoxetine concentrations and antidepressant response. *Ther Drug Monit*. 1989;11:165-170.

143. Kerr BM, Thummel KE, Wurden CJ, et al. Human liver carbamazepine metabolism. Role of CYP3A4 and CYP-2C8 in 10,11-epoxide formation. *Biochem Pharmacol*. 1994;47:1969-1979.

144. Ketter TA, Flockhart DA, Post RM, et al. The emerging role of cytochrome P450 3A in psychopharmacology. *J Clin Psychopharmacol*. 1995;15:387-398.

145. Ketter TA, Post RM, Worthington K. Principles of clinically important drug interactions with carbamazepine. Part I and Part II. *J Clin Psychopharmacol*. 1991;11:198-203, 306-313.

146. Kragh-Sorensen P, Overo KF, Peterson OL, Jensen K, Parnas W. The kinetics of citalopram: single and multiple dose studies in man. *Acta Pharmacol et Toxicol*. 1981;48: 53-60.

147. Krishna D, Klotz U. Extrahepatic metabolism of drugs in humans. *Clin Pharmacokinet*. 1994;26:144-160.

148. Kuhn R. The treatment of depressive states with G-22355 (imipramine hydrochloride). *Am J Psychiatry*. 1958;115: 459-464.

149. Kunze K, Eddy AC, Gibaldi M, Trager W. Metabolic enantiomeric interactions: the inhibition of human (S)-warfarin-7-hydroxylase by (R)-warfarin. *Chirality*. 1991;3:24-29.

150. Kupfer DJ. Long-term treatment of depression. *J Clin Psychiatry*. 1991;52(suppl 5):28-34.

151. Kupfer DJ, Frank E, Perel JM, et al. Five-year outcome for maintenance therapies in recurrent depression. *Arch Gen Psychiatry*. 1992;49:769-773.

152. Kupfer A, Preisig R. Pharmacogenetics of *p*-mephenytoin: a new drug hydroxylation polymorphism in man. *Eur J Clin Pharmacol*. 1984;26:753-759.

153. Kurtz DL, Bergstrom RF, Goldberg MJ, Cerimale BJ. Drug interation between sertraline and desipramine or imipramine. *J Clin Pharmacol*. 1994;34:1009-1033. Abstract.

154. Laborit H, Huguenard P, Alluaume R. Un nouveau stabilisateur vegetatif, le 4560 RP. *Presse Med*. 1952; 60:206-208.

155. Lader M, Melhuish A, Freka G, Fredericson, OK, Christensen V. The effects of citalopram in single and repeated doses and with alcohol on physiological and psychological measures in healthy subjects. *Eur J Clin Pharmacol*. 1986;31:183-190.

156. Lane R, Baldwin D, Preskorn S. The SSRIs: advantages, disadvantages and differences. *J Psychopharmacol*. 1995; 9(suppl):163-178.

157. Lasher TA, Fleishaker JC, Steenwyk RC, Antal EJ. Pharmacokinetic pharmacodynamic evaluation of the combined administration of alprazolam and fluoxetine. *Psychopharmacol*. 1991;104:323-327.

158. Laursen AL, Mikkelsen PL, Rasmussen S, le Fevre Honore P. Paroxetine in the treatment of depression—a randomized comparison with amitriptyline. *Acta Psychiatr Scand*. 1985;71:249-255.

159. Lemberger L, Bergstrom RF, Wolen RL, Farid NA, Enas GG, Aronoff GR. Fluoxetine: clinical pharmacology and physiologic disposition. *J Clin Psychiatry*. 1985;46:14-19.

160. Lemberger L, Rowe H, Bosomworth JC, Tenbarge JB, Bergstrom RF.The effect of fluoxetine on the pharmacokinetics and psychomotor responses of diazepam. *Clin Pharmacol Ther*. 1988;43:412-419.

161. Lemoine A, Gautier JC, Azoulay D, et al. Major pathway of imipramine metabolism is catalyzed by cytochromes P-450 1A2 and P-450 3A4 in human liver. *Mol Pharmacol*. 1993;43:827-832.

162. Lewis R, Trager W, Chan K, et al. Warfarin: stereo-chemical aspects of its metabolism and the interaction with phenylbutazone. *J Clin Invest*. 1974;53:1607-1617.

163. Lin L, Yang F, Ye Z, et al. Case-control study of cigarette smoking and primary hepatoma in an aflatoxin-endemic region of China: a protective effect. *Pharmacogenetics*. 1991;1:79-85.

164. Lingjaerde O, Bratfos O, Bratlid T, Havg JO. A double-blind comparison of zimelidine and desipramine in endogenous depression. *Acta Psychiatr Scand*. 1983;68:22-30.

165. Litovitz TL, Holm KC, Clancy C, Schmitz BF, Clark LR, Oderda GM. 1992 annual report of the American Association of Poison Control Centers Toxic Exposures Surveillance System. *Am J Emerg Med*. 1993;11:494-555.

166. Lund J, Lomholt B, Fabricius J, Christensen JA, Bechgaard E. Paroxetine: pharmacokinetics, tolerance and depletion of blood 5-HT in man. *Acta Pharmacol et Toxicol*. 1979; 44:289-295.

167. Lundmark J, Scheel K, Thomsen I, Fjord-Larsen T, et al. Paroxetine: pharmacokinetic and antidepressant effect in the elderly. *Acta Psychiatr Scand*. 1989;80(suppl 350):76-80.

168. Madsen H, Nielsen KK, Brøsen K. Imipramine metabolism in relation to the sparteine and mephenytoin oxidation polymorphisms—a population study. *Br J Clin Pharmacol*. 1995;39:433-439.

169. Marder SR, Meibach RC. Risperidone in the treatment of schizophrenia. *Am J Psychiatry*. 1994;151:825-835.

170. Marsden CA, Tyrer P, Casey P, Seivewright N. Changes in human whole blood 5-hydroxytryptamine (5-HT) and platelet 5-HT uptake during treatment with paroxetine, a selective 5-HT uptake inhibitor. *J Psychopharmacol*. 1987;1:244-250.

171. Mellstrom B, Bertilsson L, Sawe J, Schulz H, Sjoqvist F. *E*- and *Z*-hydroxylation of nortriptyline: relationship to polymorphic debrisoquine hydroxylation. *Clin Pharmacol Ther*. 1981;30:189-193.

172. Miles MV, Tennison MB. Erythromycin effects on multiple-dose carbamazepine kinetics. *Ther Drug Monit*. 1989;11:47-52.

173. Milne RJ, Goa KL. Citalopram: a review of its pharmacodynamic and pharmacokinetic properties, and therapeutic potential in depressive illness. *Drugs*. 1991;41:450-477.

174. Montgomery SA. Selecting the optimum therapeutic dose of serotonin reuptake inhibitors: studies with citalopram. *Intl Clin Psychopharmacol*. 1995;10(suppl 1):23-27.

9

175. Montgomery SA, Dufour H, Brion S, et al. The prophylactic efficacy of fluoxetine in unipolar depression. *Br J Psychiatry*. 1988;153(suppl 3):69-76.

176. Montgomery SA, Evans R. Relapse prevention with antidepressants. *Nord J Psychiatry*. 1993;47(suppl 30):83-88.

177. Montgomery SA, Pedersen V, Tanghoj P, Rasmussen C, Rioux P. The optimal dosing regimen for citalopram—a meta-analysis of nine placebo-controlled studies. *Intl Clin Psychopharmacol*. 1994;9(suppl 1):35-40.

178. Montgomery SA, Rasmussen JG, Lyby K, Connor P, Tanghoj P. Dose response relationship of citalopram 20 mg, citalopram 40 mg and placebo in the treatment of moderate and severe depression. *Intl Clin Psychopharmacol*. 1992;6(suppl 5):65-70.

179. Montgomery SA, Rasmussen JG, Tanghoj P. A 24-week study of 20 mg citalopram, 40 mg citalopram and placebo in the prevention of relapse of major depression. *Intl Clin Psychopharmacol*. 1993;8:181-188.

180. Murray M. Mechanisms of the inhibition of cytochrome P-450-mediated drug oxidation by therapeutic agents. *Drug Metabolism Reviews*. 1987;18:55-81.

181. Nakachi K, Imai K, Hayashi S, Watanabe J, Kawajiri K. Genetic susceptibility to squamous cell carcinoma of the lung in relation to cigarette smoking dose. *Cancer Res*. 1991;51:5177-5180.

182. Nathan RS, Perel JM, Pollock BG, Kupfer DJ. The role of neuropharmacologic selectivity in antidepressant action: fluvoxamine versus desipramine. *J Clin Psychiatry*. 1990; 51:367-372.

183. Nebert DW. Proposed role of drug-metabolizing enzymes: regulation of steady-state levels of the ligands that effect growth, homeostatis, differentiation, and neuroendocrine functions. *Mol Endocrinol*. 1991;5:1203-1214.

184. Nebert DW, Adesnik M, Coon MJ, et al. The P450 gene superfamily: recommended nomenclature. *DNA*. 1987;6:1-11.

185. Nebert DW, Gonzalez FJ. P450 genes: structure, evolution and regulation. *Ann Rev Biochem*. 1987;56:945-993.

186.   Nebert DW, Nelson DR, Feyereisen R. Evolution of the cytochrome P450 genes. *Xenobiotica.* 1989;19:1149-1160.

187.   Nelson DR, Kamataki T, Waxman DJ, et al. The P450 superfamily: update on new sequences, gene mapping, accession numbers, early trivial names of enzymes and nomenclature. *DNA Cell Biol.* 1993;12:1-51.

188.   Nierenberg AA, Cole JO. Antidepressant adverse drug reactions. *J Clin Psychiatry.* 1991;52(suppl):40-47.

189.   Norman TR, Gupta RK, Burrows GD, Parker G, Judd FK. Relationship between antidepressant response and plasma concentrations of fluoxetine and norfluoxetine. *Intl Clin Psychopharmacol.* 1993;8:25-29.

190.   Nystrom C, Hallstrom T. Double-blind comparison between serotonin and adrenaline reuptake blocker in the treatment of depressed outpatients: clinical aspects. *Acta Psychiatr Scand.* 1985;72:6-15.

191.   Nystrom C, Hallstrom T, et al. Comparison between serotonin and adrenaline reuptake blocker in the treatment of depressed outpatients: a crossover study. *Acta Psychiatr Scand.* 1987;75:377-382.

192.   Ohmori S, Takeda S, Rikihisa T, Kiuchi M, Kanakubo Y, Kitada M. Studies on cytochrome P450 resonsible for oxidative metabolism of imipramine in human liver microsomes. *Biol Pharm Bull.* 1993;16:571-575.

193.   Orzechowska-Juzwenko K, Wiela A, Cieslinska A, Roszkowska E. Metabolic efficiency of the liver in patients with breast cancer as determined by pharmacokinetics of phenazone. *Cancer.* 1987;59:1607-1610.

194.   Otton SV, Ball SE, Cheung SW, Inaba T, Sellers EM. Comparative inhibition of the polymorphic enzyme CYP2D6 by venlafaxine and other 5HT uptake inhibitors. *Clin Pharm Therap.* 1994;55:141.

195.   Otton SV, Inaba T, Kalow W. Inhibition of sparteine oxidation in human liver by tricyclic antidepressants and other drugs. *Life Sci.* 1983;32:795-800.

196.   Otton SV, Wu D, Joffe RT, Cheung SW, Sellers EM. Inhibition by fluoxetine of cytochrome P-450 2D6 activity. *Clin Pharm Therap.* 1993;53:401-409.

215

197. Overo KF. Preliminary studies of the kinetics of citalopram in man. *Eur J Clin Pharmacol.* 1978;14:69-73.

198. Overmars H, Scherpenisse PM, Post LC. Fluvoxamine maleate: metabolism in man. *Eur J Drug Metab Pharmacokinet.* 1983;8:269-280.

199. Palmer KJ, Benfield P. Fluvoxamine: an overview of its pharmacological properties and review of its therapeutic potential in nondepressive disorders. *CNS Drugs.* 1994; 1:57-87.

200. Pato MT, Murphy DL, DeVane CL. Sustained plasma concentrations of fluoxetine and/or norfluoxetine four and eight weeks after fluoxetine discontinuation. *J Clin Psychopharmacol.* 1991;11:224-225.

201. Pearson HJ. Interaction of fluoxetine with carbamazepine. *J Clin Psychiatry.*1990;51:126.

202. Perel JM, Shostak M, Gann E, Kantor SJ, Glassman AH. Pharmacodynamics of imipramine and clinical outcome in depressed patients. In: Gottschalk LA, Merlis S, eds. *Pharmacokinetics of Psychoactive Drugs.* New York, NY: Spectrum Publications; 1976:229-241.

203. Perucca E, Gatti G, Cipolla G, et al. Inhibition of diazepam metabolism by fluvoxamine: a pharmacokinetic study in normal volunteers. *Clin Pharmacol Ther.* 1994;56:471-476.

204. Perucca E, Gatti G, Spina E. Clinical pharmacokinetics of fluvoxamine. *Clin Pharmacokinet.* 1994;27:175-190.

205. Pfandi B, Morike K, Winne D, Schareck W, Breyer-Pfaff U. Steroselective inhibition of nortriptyline hydroxylation in man by quinidine. *Xenobiotica.* 1992;22:721-730.

206. Pirmohamed M, Kitteringham NR, Breckenridge AM, Park BK. The effect of enzyme induction on the cytochrome P450 mediated bioactivation of carbamazipine by mouse liver microsomes. *Biochem Pharmacol.* 1992;44:2307-2314.

207. Pirmohamed M, Kitteringham NR, Guenther TM, Breckenridge AM, Park BK. An investigation of the formation of cytotoxic protein-reactive and stable metabolites

from carbamazepine *in vitro*. *Biochem Pharmacol*. 1992; 43:1675-1682.

208. Pirmohamed M, Williams D, Madden S, Templeton E, Park BK. Metabolism and bioactivation of clozapine by human liver *in vitro*. *J Pharm Exp Therap*. 1995;272:984-990.

209. Pollock B. Recent developments in drug metabolism of relevance to psychiatrists. *Harvard Rev Psychiatry*. 1994; 2:204-213.

210. Preskorn SH. Antidepressant drug selection: criteria and options. *J Clin Psychiatry*. 1994;55(suppl A):6-221.

211. Preskorn SH. Comparison of the tolerability of bupropion, fluoxetine, imipramine, nefazodone, paroxetine, sertraline and venlafaxine. *J Clin Psychiatry*. 1995;56(suppl 6):12-21.

212. Preskorn SH, Burke M, Harvey A, Carmichael C. Polypharmacy in psychiatry. Presented at the 129th NCDEU meeting; May 28-31, 1996; Boca Raton, Fla.

213. Preskorn SH. Pharmacokinetics of antidepressants: why and how they are relevant to treatment. *J Clin Psychiatry*. 1993;54(suppl 9):14-34.

214. Preskorn SH. Should bupropion dosage be adjusted based upon therapeutic drug monitoring? *Psychopharmacol Bull*. 1991;27:637-643.

215. Preskorn SH. Should rational drug development in psychiatry target more than one mechanism of action in a single molecule? *Intl Rev Psychiatry*. 1995;7:17-28.

216. Preskorn SH. Sudden death and tricyclic antidepressants (TCAs): a rare adverse event linked to high TCA plasma levels. *Nord J Psychiatry*. 1993;47(suppl 30):49-55.

217. Preskorn SH. Targeted pharmacotherapy in depression management: comparative pharmacokinetics of fluoxetine, paroxetine and sertraline. *Intl Clin Psychopharmacol*. 1994;9(suppl 3):13-19.

218. Preskorn SH. What is the message in the alphabet soup of cytochrome P450 enzymes? *J Prac Psychiatry Behavioral Hlth*. 1995;1:237-240.

9

219. Preskorn SH, Alderman J, Chung M, Harrison W, Messig M, Harris S. Pharmacokinetics of desipramine coadministered with sertraline or fluoxetine. *J Clin Psychopharmacol*. 1994;14:90-98.

220. Preskorn SH, Burke M. Somatic therapy for major depressive disorder: selection of an antidepressant. *J Clin Psychiatry*. 1992;53(suppl 9):5-18.

221. Preskorn SH, Fast GA. Therapeutic drug monitoring for antidepressants: efficacy, safety and cost effectiveness. *J Clin Psychiatry*. 1991;52(suppl 6):23-33.

222. Preskorn SH, Fast GA. Tricyclic antidepressant-induced seizures and plasma drug concentration. *J Clin Psychiatry*. 1992;53:160-162.

223. Preskorn SH, Harvey A. Biochemical and clinical dose-response curves with sertaline. *Clin Pharmacol Ther*. 1996; 59:180.

224. Preskorn SH, Harvey AT, Stanga C. Drug interactions: how to understand them and their role in patient care. In: Rush AJ, ed. *Current Review of Mood Disorders*. 1996. In press.

225. Preskorn SH, Irwin HA. Toxicity of tricyclic antidepressants—kinetics, mechanism, intervention: a review. *J Clin Psychiatry*. 1982;43:151-156.

226. Preskorn SH, Janicak PG, Davis JM, Ayd FJ. Advances in the pharmacotherapy of depressive disorders. In: Janicak PG, ed. *Principles and Practices of Psychopharmacotherapy*. Baltimore, Md: Williams and Wilkins; 1995:4.

227. Preskorn SH, Jerkovich GS. Central nervous system toxicity of tricyclic antidepressants: phenomenology, course, risk factors and the role of therapeutic drug monitoring. *J Clin Psychopharmacol*. 1990;10:88-95.

228. Preskorn SH, Jerkovich GS, Beber JH, Widener P. Therapeutic drug monitoring of tricyclic antidepressants: a standard of care issue. *Psychopharmacol Bull*. 1989;25:281-284.

229. Preskorn SH, Lane RM. Sertraline 50 mg daily: the optimal dose in the treatment of depression. *Intl Clin Psychopharmacol*. 1995;10:129-141.

230. Preskorn SH, Mac DS. The implication of concentration/response studies of tricyclic antidepressants for psychiatric research and practice. *Psychiatric Develop*. 1984;2:201-222.

231. Preskorn SH, Magnus RD. Inhibition of hepatic P450 isoenzymes by serotonin selective reuptake inhibitors: *in vitro* and *in vivo* findings and their implications for patient care. *Psychopharmacol Bull*. 1994;30:251-259.

232. Preskorn SH, Silkey B, Beber J, Dorey C. Antidepressant response and plasma concentrations of fluoxetine. *Ann Clin Psychiatry*. 1991;3:147-151.

233. Prien RF, Kupfer DJ. Continuation drug therapy for major depressive episodes: how long should it be maintained? *Am J Psychiatry*. 1986;143:18-23.

234. Raghoebar M, Roseboom H. Kinetics of fluvoxamine in special populations. Poster presented at Symposium on Variability in Pharmacokinetics and Drug Response; October 3-5, 1988; Gothenburg, Germany.

235. Rasmussen BB, Maenpaa J, Pelkonen O, et al. Selective serotonin reuptake inhibitors and theophylline metabolism in human liver microsomes: potent inhibition by fluvoxamine. *Br J Clin Pharmacol*. 1995;39:151-159.

236. Ray WA, Griffin MR, Schaffner W, Baugh DK, Melton LJ III. Psychotropic drug use and the risk of hip fracture. *N Engl J Med*. 1987;316:363-369.

237. Reimherr FW, Chouinard G, Cohn CK, et al. Antidepressant efficacy of sertraline: a double-blind, placebo- and amitriptyline-controlled, multicenter comparison study in outpatients with major depression. *J Clin Psychiatry*. 1990;51(suppl B):18-27.

238. Rettie AE, Korzekwa KR, Kunze KL, et al. Hydroxylation of warfarin by human cDNA-expressed cytochrome P-450: a role for P-4502C9 in the etiology of (S)-warfarin-drug interactions. *Chem Res Toxicol*. 1992;5:54-59.

239. Richelson E. Pharmacology of antidepressants—characteristics of the ideal drug. *Mayo Clin Proc*. 1994;69:1069-1081.

9

240. Robert P, Montgomery SA. Citalopram in doses of 20-60 mg is effective in depression relapse prevention: a placebo-controlled 6-month study. *Intl Clin Psychopharmacol.* 1995;10(suppl 1):29-35.

241. Robertson MM,Trimble MR. Depressive illness in patients with epilepsy: a review. *Epilepsia.* 1983;24(suppl 2):109-116.

242. Rochat B, Amey M, Baumann P. Analysis of enantiomers of citalopram and its demethylated metabolites in plasma of depressive patients using chiral reverse-phase liquid chromatography. *Therap Drug Monit.* 1995;17:273-279.

243. Ronfeld RA, Tremaine LM, Wilner KD, Henry EB. Evaluation of the pharmacokinetic properties of sertraline and desmethylsertraline in elderly and young normal volunteers. *Clin Pharmacokinet.* In press.

244. Roose SP, Glassman AH, Attia E, Woodring S. Comparative efficacy of selective serotonin reuptake inhibitors and tricyclics in the treatment of melanchia. *Am J Psychiatry.* 1994;151:1735-1739.

245. Rowe H, Carmichael R, Lemberger L. The effect of fluoxetine on warfarin metabolism in the rat and man. *Life Sci.* 1978;23:807-812.

246. Schenker S, Bergstrom RF, Wolen RL, Lemberger L. Fluoxetine disposition and elimination in cirrhosis. *Clin Pharmacol Ther.* 1988;44:353-359.

247. Schmider J, Greenblatt DJ, von Moltke LL, Harmatz JS, Shader RI. *N*-demethylation of amitriptyline *in vitro*: role of cytochrome P450 3A (CYP3A) isoforms and effect of metabolic inhibitors. *J Pharmacol Exp Ther.* 1995;275:592-597.

248. Series HG. Drug treatment of depression in medically ill patients. *J Psychosom Res.* 1992;36:1-16.

249. Shader RI, Greenblatt DJ, von Moltke LL. Fluoxetine inhibition of phenytoin metabolism. *J Clin Psychopharmacol.* 1994;14:375-376. Editorial.

250. Shank RP, Vaught JL, Pelley KA, Setler PE, McComsey DF, Maryanoff BE. McN-5652: a highly potent inhibitor of

serotonin uptake. *J Pharm Exp Therap.* 1988;247:1032-1038.

251.   Shaw CA, Sullivan JT, Kadlec KE, Kaplan HL, Naranjo CA, Sellers EM. Ethanol interactions with serotonin uptake selective and nonselective antidepressants: fluoxetine and amitriptyline. *Human Psychopharmacol.* 1989;4:113-120.

252.   Sindrup SH, Brøsen K, Gram LF. Pharmacokinetics of the selective serotonin reuptake inhibitor paroxetine: non-linearity and relation to the sparteine oxidation polymorphism. *Clin Pharm Ther.* 1992;51:288-295.

253.   Sindrup SH, Brøsen K, Gram LF, et al. The relationship between paroxetine and the sparteine oxidation polymorphism. *Clin Pharmacol Ther.* 1992;51:278-287.

254.   Sindrup SH, Brøsen K, Hansen MG, Aaes-Jorgensen T, Overo KF, Gram LF. Pharmacokinetics of citalopram in relation to the sparteine and the mephenytoin oxidation polymorphisms. *Ther Drug Monit.* 1993;15:11-17.

255.   Sjoerdsma T, Palfregman A. History of serotonin. In: Peroutka S, Whitaker-Azmitia P, eds. *Neuropharmacology of Serotonin.* New York, NY: Annals of the New York Academy of Science; 1990;600:2-9.

256.   Skjelbo E, Brøsen K. Inhibitors of imipramine metabolism by human liver microsomes. *Br J Clin Pharmacol.* 1992; 34:256-261.

257.   Skjelbo E, Brøsen K, Hallas J, Gram LF. The mephenytoin oxidation polymorphism is partially responsible for the *N*-demethylation of imipramine. *Clin Pharm Therap.* 1991; 49:18-23.

258.   Smith SJ. Cardiovascular toxicity of antihistamines. *Otolaryngol Head Neck Surg.* 1994;111:348-354.

259.   Sommi RW, Crismon ML. Bowden CL. Fluoxetine: a serotonin-specific second-generation antidepressant. *Pharmacotherapy.* 1987;7:1-15.

260.   Sperber AD. Toxic interaction between fluvoxamine and sustained release theophylline in an 11-year-old boy. *Drug Safety.* 1991;6:460-462.

9

261. Spina E, Avenoso A, Pollicino AM, Caputi AP, Fazio A, Pisani F. Carbamazepine coadministration with fluoxetine or fluvoxamine. *Ther Drug Monit.* 1993;15:247-250.

262. Spina E, Birgersson C, von Bahr C, et al. Phenotypic consistency in hydroxylation of desmethylimipramine and debrisoquine in healthy subjects and in human liver microsomes. *Clin Pharm Therap.* 1984;36:677-682.

263. Spina E, Pollicino AM, Avenoso A, Campo GM, Perucca E, Caputi AP. Effect of fluvoxamine on the pharmacokinetics of imipramine and desipramine in healthy subjects. *Ther Drug Monit.* 1993;15:243-246.

264. Sproule BA, Otton SV, Cheung SW, Zhong XH, Romach MK, Sellers EM. Does sertraline inhibit CYP 2D6 after chronic dosing? *Clin Pharm Therap.* 1995;57:151.

265. Steiner E, Bertilsson L, Sawe J, Bertling I, Sjoqvist F. Polymorphic debrisoquine hydroxylation in 757 Swedish subjects. *Clin Pharm Therap.* 1988;44:431-435.

266. Sternbach H. The serotonin syndrome. *Am J Psychiatry.* 1991;148:705-713.

267. Stevens JC, Wrighton SA. Interaction of the enantiomers of fluoxetine and norfluoxetine with human liver cytochromes P450. *J Pharm Exp Therap.* 1993;266:964-971.

268. Swims MP. Potential terfenadine-fluoxetine interaction. *Ann Pharmacotherapy.* 1993;17:1404.

269. Tasker TCG, Kaye CM, Zussman BD, Link CGG. Paroxetine plasma levels: lack of correlation with efficacy or adverse events. *Acta Psychiatr Scand.* 1989;80(suppl 350): 152-155.

270. Thomson AH, McGovern EM, Bennie P, Caldwell G, Smith M. Interaction between fluvoxamine and theophylline. *Pharmaceutical J.* 1992;1:137.

271. Tork I. Anatomy of the serotonergic system. In: Peroutka S, Whitaker-Azmitia P, eds. *Neuropharmacology of Serotonin.* New York, NY: Annals of the New York Academy of Science; 1990;600:9-35.

272. Torok-Both GA, Baker GB, Coutts RT, McKenna KF, Aspeslet LJ. Simultaneous determination of fluoxetine and

norfluoxetine enantiomers in biological samples by gas chromatography with electron-capture detection. *J Chromatography*. 1992;579:99-106.

273.   Tremaine LM, Wilner KD, Henry EB, Ronfeld RA. Absence of a biologically meaningful effect of sertraline on the pharmacokinetics and protein binding of tolbutamide. *Clin Pharmacokinet*. In press.

274.   van Harten J. Clinical pharmacokinetics of selective serotonin reuptake inhibitors. *Clin Pharmacokinet*. 1993;24:203-220.

275.   van Harten J, Stevens LA, Raghoebar M, Holland RL, Wesnes K, Cournot A. Fluvoxamine does not interact with alcohol or potentiate alcohol-related impairment of cognitive function. *Clin Pharmacol Ther*. 1992;52:427-435.

276.   von Moltke LL, Greenblatt DJ, Cotreau-Bibbo MM, Duan SX, Harmatz JS, Shader RI. Inhibition of desipramine hydroxylation *in vitro* by serotonin-reuptake-inhibitor antidepressants, and by quinidine and ketoconazole: a model system to predict drug interactions *in vivo*. *J Pharm Exp Therap*. 1994;268:1278-1283.

277.   von Moltke LL, Greenblatt DJ, Cotreau-Bibbo M, Harmatz J, Shader R. Inhibitors of alprazolam metabolism *in vitro*: effect of serotonin reuptake inhibitor antidepressants, ketoconazole and quinidine. *Br J Clin Pharmacol*. 1994;38:23-31.

278.   von Moltke LL, Greenblatt DJ, Court MH, et al. Inhibition of alprazolam and desipramine hydroxylation *in vitro* by paroxetine and fluvoxamine: comparison with other selective serotonin reuptake inhibitor antidepressants. *J Clin Psychopharm*. 1995;15:125-131.

279.   von Moltke LL, Greenblatt DJ, Duan SX, Harmatz JS, Shader RI. *In vitro* prediction of the terfenadine-ketoconazole pharmacokinetic interaction. *J Clin Pharmacol*. 1994;34:1222-1227.

280.   Walker PW, Cole JO, Gardner EA, et al. Improvement in fluoxetine-associated sexual dysfunction in patients switched to bupropion. *J Clin Psychiatry*. 1993;54:459-465.

9

281. Warrington SJ. Clinical implications of the pharmacology of sertraline. *Intl Clin Psychopharmacol*. 1991;6(suppl 2): 11-21.

282. Watkins PB. Drug metabolism by cytochromes P450 in the liver and small bowel. *Gastroenterol Clin N Am*. 1992;21: 511-526.

283. Wernicke JF, Dunlop SR, Dornseif BE, Bosomworth JC, Humbert M. Low dose fluoxetine therapy for depression. *Psychopharmacol Bull*. 1988;24:183-188.

284. Wernicke JF, Dunlop SR, Dornseif BE, Zerbe RL. Fixed dose fluoxetine therapy for depression. *Psychopharmacol Bull*. 1987;23:164-168.

285. Wilde MI, Plosker GL, Benfield P. Fluvoxamine: an updated review of its pharmacology and therapeutic use in depressive illness. *Drugs*. 1993;46:895-924.

286. Wilkinson G, Guengerich FP, Branch RA. Genetic polymorphism of *S*-mephenytoin hydroxylation. *Pharmacol Ther*. 1989;43:53-76.

287. Wilner KD, Apseloff G, Gerber N, Henry EB, Lazar JD, Tremaine LM. Absence of a biologically meaningful effect of sertraline on the pharmacodynamics and protein binding of warfarin. *Clin Pharmacokinet*. In press.

288. Wilner KD, Preskorn SH. The pharmacokinetics of sertraline. *Clin Pharmacokinet*. In press.

289. Wolf ME, Bukowski ED, Conran J, et al. Polypharmacy: a problem of the decade of the nineties. American Psychiatric Association, 148th annual meeting; May 20-25, 1995; Miami, Fla. Abstract.

290. Wong DT, Bymaster FP, Reid LR, Mayle DA, Krushinski JH, Robertson DW. Norfluoxetine enantiomers as inhibitors of serotonin uptake in rat brain. *Neuropsychopharmacology*. 1993;8:337-344.

291. Wong DT, Fuller RW, Robertson DW. Fluoxetine and its two enantiomers as selective serotonin uptake inhibitors. *Acta Pharm Nord*. 1990;2:171-180.

292. Wood K, Swade C, Abou-Saleh M, Milln P, Coppen A. Drug plasma levels and platelet 5-HT uptake inhibition during long-term treatment with fluvoxamine or lithium in patients with affective disorders. *Br J Clin Pharmacol*. 1983;15(suppl 3):365S-368S.

293. Woods DJ, Coulter DM, Pillans P. Interaction of phenytoin and fluoxetine. *N Z Med J*. 1994;107:19.

294. Yasumori T, Nagata K, Yang SK, et al. Cytochrome P450 mediated metabolism of diazepam in human and rat: involvement of human CYP2C in *N*-demethylation in the substrate concentration-dependent manner. *Pharmacogenetics*. 1993;3:291-301.

295. Yun CH, Okerholm RA, Guengerich FP. Oxidation of the antihistaminic drug terfenadine in human liver microsomes. Role of cytochrome P-450 3A(4) in *N*-dealkylation and *C*-hydroxylation. *Drug Metabolism and Disposition Diol Fate Chem*. 1993;21:403-409.

296. Zajecka J, Fawcett J, Schaff M, et al. The role of serotonin in sexual dysfunction: fluoxetine-associated orgasm dysfunction. *J Clin Psychiatry*. 1991;52:66-68.

297. Zimmermann M, Duruz H, Guinand O, et al. Torsades de pointes after treatment with terfenadine and ketoconazole. *Eur Heart J*. 1992;13:1002-1003.

298. Zussman BD, Davie CC, Fowles SE, et al. Sertraline, like other SSRIs, is a significant inhibitor of desipramine metabolism *in vivo*. *Br J Clin Pharmacol*. 1995;39:550-551.

299. von Moltke LL, Greenblatt DJ, Duan SX, Schmider J, Narmatz JS, Shader RI. *In vitro* biotransformation of phenacetin to acetaminophen. *Clin Pharm Therap*. 1996;59:175.

300. Centurrino F, Baldessarini RJ, Kando JC, Frankenburg FR, Volpicelli SA, Flood JG. Clozapine and metabolites: concentrations in serum and clinical findings during treatment of chronically psychotic patients. *J Clin Psychopharmacol*. 1994;14:119-125.

301. Nemeroff CB, DeVane CL, Pollock BG. Newer antidepressants and the cytochrome P450 system. *Am J Psychiatry*. 1996;153:311-320.

9

302. DeVane CL. Pharmacokinetics of the newer antidepressants: clinical relevance. *Am J Med*. 1994;97(suppl 6A): 13S-23S.

303. Fleishaker JC, Hulst LK. A pharmacokinetic and pharmacodynamic evaluation of the combined administration of alprazolam and fluoxetine. *Eur J Clin Pharmacol*. 1994; 46:35-39.

304. Greenblatt DJ, Preskorn SH, Cotreau MM, Horst WD, Harmatz JS. Fluoxetine impairs clearance of alprazolam but not of clonazepam. *Clin Pharmacol Ther*. 1992;52:479-486.

305. Olkkola KT, Aranko K, Luurila H, et al. A potentially hazardous interaction between erythromycin and midazolam. *Clin Pharmacol Ther*. 1993;53:298-305.

306. Varhe A, Olkkola KT, Neuvonen PJ. Oral triazolam is potentially hazardous to patients receiving systemic antimycotics ketoconazole and itraconazole. *Clin Pharmacol Ther*. 1994;56:601-607.

10 Appendix

As discussed in Section 8, the *in vitro* inhibition constant (K_i) is not the sole determinant of whether a drug will produce a clinically meaningful or even detectable *in vivo* effect on a cytochrome P450 (CYP) enzyme under clinically relevant dosing conditions. Instead, it is only one factor in the equation:

Equation 1:

Magnitude of Effect	=	Affinity for Site of Action × Drug Concentration at Site of Action × Underlying Biology of Patient

For this reason, the K_i has relatively limited value without knowing or at least having a reasonable estimate of the concentration of the potential inhibitor at the site of action (eg, the CYP enzyme). Parenthetically, the location of the relevant CYP enzyme may be extrahepatic in some instances, such as in the gut wall in the case of the inhibition of the first pass metabolism of terfenadine.

Although some reviews have attempted to rank or list drugs as enzyme inhibitors based on primarily *in vitro* data or isolated case reports of possible interactions,[2] this approach does not convey to the clinician whether an interaction is likely to occur in clinical practice or to what extent. Answers to these questions require knowing the concentration of the drug that will occur under clinically relevant dosing conditions as well as the K_i.

This appendix is for the reader who would like more background on this issue from a mathematical perspective, but is not intended to be a rigorous mathematical treatise on the subject. This discussion is relevant to any drug or class of drugs capable of inhibiting a CYP enzyme; however, it will use the SSRIs as the example since they are the subject of this book. The reader who would like further discussion of these matters is referred to the work of Segel[3] and von Moltke and colleagues.[4]

For this discussion, we must recall some basic principles of biochemistry, specifically enzymology. The relationship between the inhibition of an enzyme caused by a competitive inhibitor and the concentration of the inhibitor is expressed by the equation:

Equation 2:

$$i = [I] / \left([I] + K_i (1 + [S] / K_m) \right)$$

where "i" is the fractional inhibition of the enzyme, [I] is the concentration of the inhibitor, K_i is the inhibition constant of the inhibitor for the enzyme, [S] is the concentration of the substrate normally biotransformed by the enzyme, and K_m is the affinity constant of that substrate for that enzyme.

If [S] is less than K_m as is the case *in vivo* for drugs with linear pharmacokinetics,then the fractional inhibition is independent of the substrate concentration and the equation reduces to:

Equation 3:

$$i = [I] / \left([I] + K_i \right)$$

Hence, to the first approximation, the fractional inhibition of the enzyme is determined by the concentration of the inhibitor directly and by the K_i of the inhibitor reciprocally. The smaller K_i is to [I], the more "i" approaches unity:

Equation 4:

$$i = [I] / [I] \text{ (when } K_i <<<< [I])$$

Equation 4 illustrates why both K_i and [I] are important when trying to determine whether a clinically meaningful degree of enzyme inhibition is likely to occur under clinically relevant dosing conditions. Parenthetically, the relative K_i's in some studies (eg, Crewe et al, 1991) can be outliers relative to the ones derived from other *in vitro* studies (Table 8.7). If the concentration of the substrate used in the study not being much less than its K_m and not reflective of what would be expected *in vivo*.

Since all of the SSRIs except possibly fluvoxamine have "active" metabolites in terms of the inhibition of specific CYP enzymes such as CYP 2D6, one must have equation 3 for the parent drug and all of its relevant metabolites when doing projections from *in vitro* work to *in vivo* reality. Parenthetically, formal *in vivo* pharmacokinetic studies measure the summed effect of the parent drug and all of the relevant metabolites at the relative concentrations that they occur under clinically relevant dosing conditions, assuming that the drug is given as it would normally be given and given for a sufficient period of time to reach steady-state conditions.

This last condition has not been true for many of the fluoxetine studies reviewed in Section 8. Instead, loading dose strategies (eg, 60 mg/day × 8 days) have commonly been used due to the long period of time that the study will have to go to reach steady-state conditions of fluoxetine and norfluoxetine. The results of such loading dose strategies may underestimate the actual effect that will occur under more clinically relevant dosing conditions for several reasons. First, norfluoxetine is more potent than fluoxetine in terms of the inhibition of some CYP enzymes such as CYP 3A3/4. Secondly, the conversion of fluoxetine to norfluoxetine takes time. Third, this conversion is inhibited by high concentrations of fluoxetine and/or norfluoxetine. Hence, such loading dose approaches may underestimate the ratio of norfluoxetine to fluoxetine that will be expected under truly steady-state conditions and thus underestimate the concentration of the more portent CYP 3A3/4 inhibitor, norfluoxetine. For these reasons, the results from the loading studies with fluoxetine must be interpreted cautiously and do not reflect the effect that will occur under steady-state conditions at at 20 mg/day, much less 60 mg/day.

The next step in trying to relate *in vitro* results to *in vivo* reality is to determine what is the relevant concentration at the CYP enzyme. The concentration of the drug in plasma is the most readily measured concentration; however, the enzyme is not in the plasma, but rather in some tissue compartments. The hepatic tissue compartment is the one which is generally most relevant to predicting whether a pharmacokinetic drug-drug interaction is likely to occur due to the inhibition of a CYP enzyme. For this reason, we need to either measure or estimate the hepatic concentration of the drug which occurs in this compartment under clinically relevant dosing conditions.

Typically, the hepatic concentration is estimated rather than directly measured. It is estimated based on measuring the plasma drug concentration of the drug and its plasma:liver partition coefficient (Table 10.1). The plasma:liver partition coefficient is empirically determined in animals and then can be confirmed in man using autopsy or surgical material.

Table 10.1 illustrates how such information can be used to estimate the relative inhibition of a specific CYP enzyme using such information. Table 10.1 compares the estimated inhibition of CYP 2D6 by 4 different SSRIs. First, the average K_i for each SSRI was calculated using the data from the 5 *in vitro* studies reported in Table 8.7. Since all 5 of these studies measured the K_i for fluoxetine but not for all the other SSRIs, the average K_i for fluoxetine was determined and used to normalize the K_i values for all the other SSRIs in terms of their relative value compared to fluoxetine. The plasma levels of the different SSRIs which would be expected under comparable antidepressant treatment conditions was then determined. The hepatic concentration of each SSRI which would be expected under such conditions was then estimated based on each drug's plasma:liver partition coefficient times their expected plasma drug concentration at steady-state under comparable antidepressant treatment conditions. These values and equation 2 above correctly predict the substantial differences in the degree of CYP2D6 inhibition which has been measured in the 11 formal *in vivo* pharmacokinetic

10

TABLE 10.1 — VARIABLES WHICH DETERMINE THE MAGNITUDE OF THE EFFECT *IN VIVO*: CYP 2D6 AS AN EXAMPLE

	Fluvoxamine	Fluoxetine	Paroxetine	Sertraline
Relative K_i	9.4	1.0	0.8	6.4
Estimated K_i (M)	8.31	0.88	0.71	5.66
Plasma concentration (nM)	164.0	512.0	135.0	66.0
Liver:water partition ratio	26.6	12.1	26.2	12.2
Liver concentration (M)	4.4	6.2	3.5	0.8
Change in desipramine* • PK studies (AUC)	14%	380% to 640%	327% to 421%	0% to 37%

* Above baseline.

AUC = Area under curve.

References: 120

studies reviewed in Section 8 on the relative effects of these SSRIs on CYP 2D6 function. As can be readily seen, a comparison using the K_i alone will lead one to erroneously conclude that there may be minimal differences between these different SSRIs with regard to the inhibition of this enzyme under clinically relevant conditions.

The next issue is how the fractional inhibition of the enzyme relates to the change in the concentration of a concomitantly administered drug which is dependent on the functional integrity of this enzyme for its clearance. In clinical practice, the term "concentration" usually refers to either a 12-hour post-dose concentration or a trough concentration (ie, the concentration immediately before the next dose of drug is given). In both instances, these concentrations are typically measured after steady-state has been attained or assumed to have been attained. A more rigorous measurement is to measure the area under the plasma concentration-time curve (AUC) under steady-state conditions. The latter approach is typically used in formal pharmacokinetic studies. Nonetheless, both approaches have been used to assess the change in the drug concentration as a function of the decrease in its clearance produced by the inhibition of the principal CYP enzyme responsible for the biotransformation necessary for the drug's elimination. The increase in the AUC with the inhibitor present (AUCi) relative to the AUC without the inhibitor present is related to the fractional inhibition of the enzyme (i) as follows:

Equation 5:

$$AUCi/AUCo = I/ \left(1\text{-}I \right)$$

As can be readily appreciated, equation 5 describes a complex hyperbolic relationship (Figure 10.1) between the fractional inhibition of the enzyme and the change in the plasma concentration of the drug whose metabolism has been inhibited. This curve approximates linearity over narrow portions of the curve. As the inhibitions increase, the increase in the plasma concentration of the affected drug increases disproportionately. This fact further explains the differences in clearance of drugs such as desipramine which are observed when fluoxetine and paroxetine are coprescribed at their usually effective minimum antidepressant doses versus citalopram, fluvoxamine, and sertraline (Table 10.1). Fluoxetine and paroxetine produce substantially more than 50% inhibition of the enzyme in contrast to the other 3 SSRIs and thus are on the rapidly ascending portion of this hyperbolic curve.

As stated at the beginning, this discussion has used the effect of the SSRIs on CYP 2D6 to illustrate the enzymological and pharmacokinetic principles relevant to understanding in greater depth the differential effects of drug-induced inhibition of CYP enzyme-

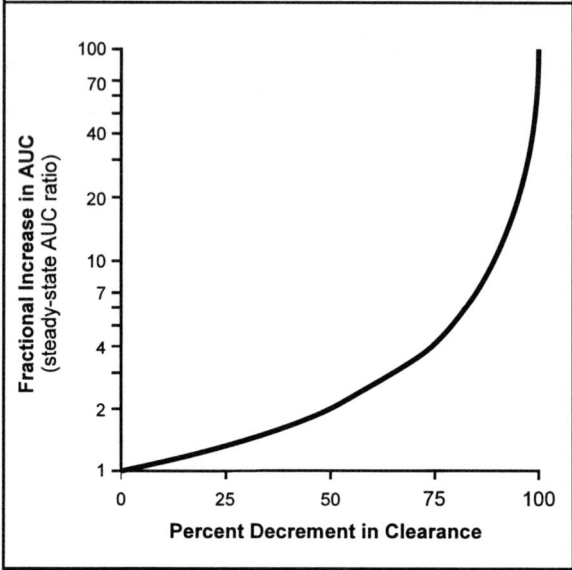

FIGURE 10.1

Fractional Increase in AUC (steady-state AUC ratio) vs. Percent Decrement in Clearance

mediated clearance of concomitantly prescribed drugs. These principles are relevant to the effects of the SSRIs on other CYP enzymes and to the effects of other drugs on the various CYP enzymes.

Using the approach explained above, *in vitro* studies can be used to screen already marketed drugs or drugs in the development for their effects on CYP enzymes and to predict using a knowledge of their K_i, the plasma drug concentration expected under clinically relevant dosing conditions and the plasma:liver partition coefficient whether a clinically meaningful change in the clearance of specific drugs can be expected if they were concomitantly administered with the potential inhibitor. Based on such *in vitro* modeling, appropriate *in vivo* studies can be done on a selective basis to confirm such predictions when such an interaction would be predicted to occur in a significant number of patients (ie, the drugs are likely to be frequently coprescribed together) and the consequences are predicted to be clinically important. The advantage of this sequential *in vitro* and then *in vivo* approach is the cost and time efficiency of doing *in vitro* rather than *in vivo* studies to screen the drugs against a full battery of CYP enzymes.

Given this discussion, readers can anticipate that they will be hearing more and more about the effects of a wide variety of drugs on CYP enzymes. This information will aid the physicians in anticipating pharmacokinetic interactions and will allow them to make appropriate treatment decisions (eg, drug selection, dose adjustments) to avoid adverse consequences of such interactions. The SSRIs and their differential effects on CYP enzymes have been a significant impetus and vehicle for educating physicians about this important advance in our knowledge.

Suggested Further Readings:

1. Harvey AT, Preskorn SH. Interactions of serotonin reuptake inhibitors with tricyclic antidepressants. *Arch Gen Psychiatry*. 1995;52:783-784.

2. Nemeroff CB, DeVane CL, Pollock BG. Newer antidepressants and the cytochrome P450 system. *Am J Psychiatry*. 1996;153: 311-320.

3. Segel I. *Enzyme Kinetics: Behavior and Analysis of Rapid Equilibrium and Steady-state Enzyme Systems*. New York, NY: J Wiley and Sons; 1975:105.

4. von Moltke LL, Greenblatt DJ, Schmider J, Harmatz JS, Shader RI. Metabolism of drugs by cytochrome P450 3A isoforms: implications for drug interactions in psychopharmacology. *Clin Pharmacokinet*. 1995;29(suppl 1):33-44.

10

TABLE 10.2 — SSRIS: BRAND NAMES BY COUNTRY

Country	Citalopram	Fluoxetine	Fluvoxamine	Paroxetine	Sertraline
Argentina	—	Animex-On Equilibrane Foxetin Neupax Saurat	—	Aropax	Zoloft
Australia	—	Prozac 20	—	Aropax	Zoloft
Austria	Seropram	Fluctine	Floxyfral	Seroxat	Tresleen
Belgium	Cipramil	Prozac	Floxyfral	Aropax Seroxat	Serlain
Brazil	—	Prozac 20 Eufor 20 Daforin	—	Aropax	Zoloft
Canada	—	Prozac	Luvox	Paxil	Zoloft
Denmark	Cipramil	Fontex Fonzac	Fevarin	Seroxat	Zoloft

Finland	Cipramil	Fontex Seronil	Fevarin	Seroxat	Zoloft
France	Cipramil	Prozac	Floxyfral	Deroxat	Zoloft
Germany	Saroten	Fluctin	Fevarin	Seroxat Tagonis	Zoloft
Greece	Seropram	Flonital Fluxadir Ladose Orthon	Dumyrox	Seroxat	—
Italy	—	Fluoxeren Prozac	Dumirox Fevarin Maveral	Sereupin Seroxat	Serad Tatig Zoloft
Mexico	—	Fluoxac Prozac	—	Aropax Paxil	Altruline
Netherlands	—	Prozac	Fevarin	Seroxat	Zoloft
Norway	Cipramil	Fontex	Fevarin	Seroxat	Zoloft

10

Country	Citalopram	Fluoxetine	Fluvoxamine	Paroxetine	Sertraline
Portugal	—	Digassim Nodepe Prozac Psipax Tuneluz	Dumyrox	—	—
South Africa	Cipramil	Prozac	Luvox	Aropax 20	Zoloft
Spain	—	Adofen Prozac Reneuron	Dumirox	Frosinor Motivan Seroxat	Aramis Besitran
Sweden	Cipramil	—	Fevarin	Seroxat	Zoloft
Switzerland	Seropram	Fluctine	Floxyfral	Deroxat	Zoloft Gladem
Turkey	—	Depreks Prozac	Faverin	—	Lustral
United Kingdom	—	Prozac	Faverin	Seroxat	Lustral
United States	—	Prozac	Luvox	Paxil	Zoloft

Index

(Page numbers in italics indicate figures;
page numbers followed by "t" indicate tables.)